Finishing Well - Finding the Joy In Dementia

Senia Owensby, CLC

ISBN 978-0-9962978-0-6

Dedication

This project is dedicated to my Mama who exemplifies a lifetime of '*Finishing Well*'. She has always been an inspiration to those in her world as she lived with simple grace and acceptance of her circumstances. Her steadfast reply to anyone who asked how she was would always be:

"I'm in awfully good shape for the shape I'm in."

Acknowledgment

This project is both a labor of love and a family affair. My husband Wayne, who has been a constant source of support as well as my sister, Peggy Whitten and I have all walked this journey with Mama together. My daughter Bambi Owensby also contributed to this work. These stories are snapshots of our life along the way. Mama, the star of this book has given greatly of herself over the course of her lifetime. Her attitude of contentment has been an inspiration to us all - I want to be like her when I grow up.

Table of contents

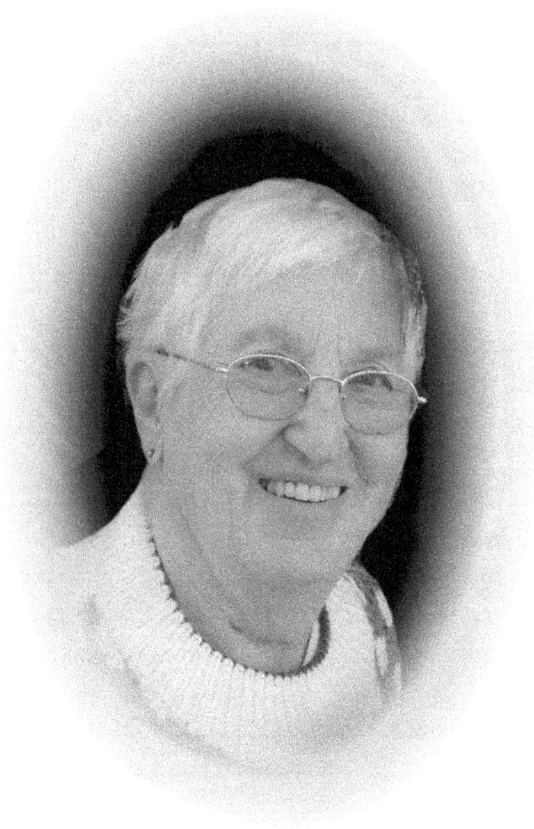

Introduction

Dementia is a tough disease. It wreaks havoc on the emotions of both loved ones and caregivers. It can often be a long trek – taking you up the hills of lost-ness and confusion, as well as down through the valley of the shadow of death.

We don't know how to fix it nor do we have all the answers, but we have walked this road with Mama who is currently in the final stage of dementia.

It is our prayer that the stories in this book will be both a help and an encouragement for your own unique journey.

"The memory of the righteous is blessed"

Proverbs 10:7

Chapter 1

The Question

"Will you promise to take care of Mama?"

Daddy's question startled me, but I quickly assured him that, of course I would. He seemed somewhat reassured by my response. Looking back, I believe that somehow he knew his time was limited, and he needed to know that Mama would be taken care of.

The question was surprising because my sister, my husband, and I were already taking care of their shopping, cooking, cleaning, and bill paying. Several times per day we administered medicine and injections, as well as handling all of the other duties required to care for parents whose abilities were diminishing.

What I hadn't considered at the time was that while we performed every physical and administrative task, Daddy was carrying a 24/7 emotional burden of love and concern for his bride of over 50 years. He was consumed with worry. Loving Mama and worrying about what would happen to her if something happened to him must have been overwhelming. I suspect Daddy lacked the energy to even notice our contribution. He suffered from Parkinson's disease and passed away a few months later due to a massive stroke.

During the early onset of dementia, I remember how heartbreaking it was to watch as Mama transitioned from a smart and witty medical professional to someone who was becoming progressively limited in her capacity to do her usual, everyday activities.

Like many others, we hadn't noticed Mama's condition at first. It was easy to excuse and explain away. Resistance to taking medicine was perceived as non-compliance, not forgetfulness. Failure to tell us what the doctor had said was perceived as unwillingness, not forgetfulness. Reluctance to eat was perceived as a lack of appetite, not forgetfulness.

It didn't begin with a bang or a diagnosis from a doctor. It didn't announce itself and take over. No, it was more like a sneaky thief. At first it seemed that something was simply odd or out of place, but then as time went on we began to put it all together: medicine not taken, meals neither prepared, nor eaten, no letters written or crossword puzzles started.

Bits and pieces of activities from all the things that are part of an everyday routine were gradually disappearing. Dementia had snuck in quietly and begun to steal away parts of Mama's life—her memories and abilities.

As time went on, we grew to learn that even though Mama couldn't do everything in the same way or manner she had in the past, there was still a lot of living ahead, and our task was to walk this journey beside her.

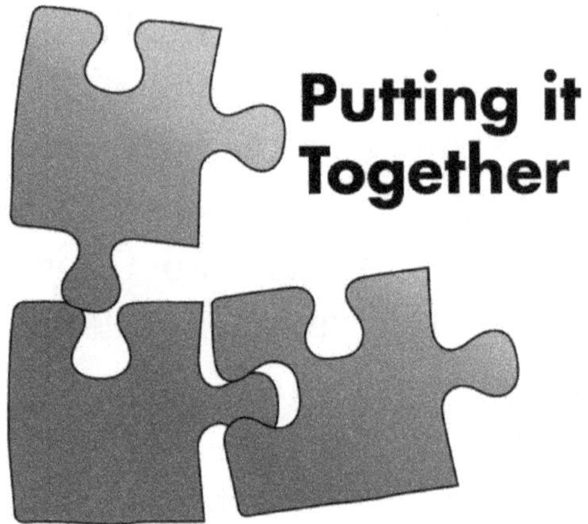
Putting it
Together

Listening is essential. *The initial awareness of dementia brings to mind several concerns and fears both spoken and unspoken. Some are deep-seated and unconscious and others are at the surface.*

Not everyone is comfortable voicing their worries. Body language speaks volumes so it is important, especially at this point, to listen to both the verbal and non-verbal messages.

Take every concern from either your loved one or other family members serious no matter how lightly they are expressed. It benefits everyone involved if you can assist in alleviating as many issues and concerns as possible, not just the issues you see as most pressing.

Some folks are not able to ask for help even when it is clearly needed. Try gently offering your assistance with critical issues in order to get the conversation started.

"The best and most beautiful things in the world cannot be seen or even touched - they must be felt with the heart."

- Hellen Keller

Chapter 2

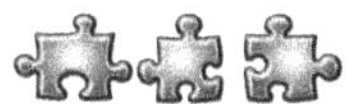

Music Connection

Music was the one constant. Music, particularly singing songs, grew in importance on our journey. Singing was always a big part of our lives; in fact, I can never remember a time when Mama didn't sing. It seemed she was always singing, especially in the car.

Every summer, while Daddy was working on his Master's Degree, we would leave for Michigan as soon as our school got out so he could begin his. Our grandparents lived in Gladstone, Michigan, which is not too far from Northern Michigan University in Marquette where Daddy attended a summer school program. So on those long drives from California to Michigan, we would sing, sing, sing.

We had sets of songs. Mama had her songs - her absolute favorite was "My Wild, Irish Rose"—but she also loved the popular songs of the day such as: "You are My Sunshine," "Bicycle Built For Two," "In the Good Old Summertime," "Red River Valley," "Let Me Call You Sweetheart," and "Que Sera, Sera." Daddy had his – which were mostly 'southern songs' like: "O Susanna," "On Top of Old Smokey," "The Old Folks at Home," and "Little Brown Jug."

We had patriotic, silly and church songs, of which included, "God Bless America," "This Land is My Land," "Mairzy Doats," "Playmate, Come out and Play With Me," "Amazing Grace," and the "Doxology."

Mama and Daddy both loved Broadway musicals and had albums of all the soundtracks of their favorites. The top of the list were the ones for which Rodgers and Hammerstein had written the music, such as: "The Sound of Music," "Oklahoma!" and "South Pacific." They also loved anything by Gilbert and Sullivan. Our two main activities during those long road trips were singing songs and spotting license plates from other states—something I'm compelled to do to this day.

Then there were songs from 'Soundies' that Daddy had bought from a catalog and had spliced together into large reels (*'Soundies' were a sort of precursors to music videos. They were produced back in the 1940's and designed for coin-operated, rear-projection machines found in bars and restaurants.*) Some of the songs from the 'Soundies' were, "Number Ten Lullaby Lane," "We're The Couple in the Castle," "Sailor with the Navy Blue Eyes," "It's a Great Day for the Irish," and "Molly Malone".

We didn't watch much TV in those days. Our evening entertainment often began with the sound of Daddy in the kitchen pouring popcorn into a pan. That was the signal we would soon be viewing reels of music videos projected onto a screen in the living room.

Since Daddy used a regular 16mm front projector, all of the song titles and credits displayed backwards on the screen and everyone in the videos was left-handed. It was great fun reading the words backwards and learning the songs.

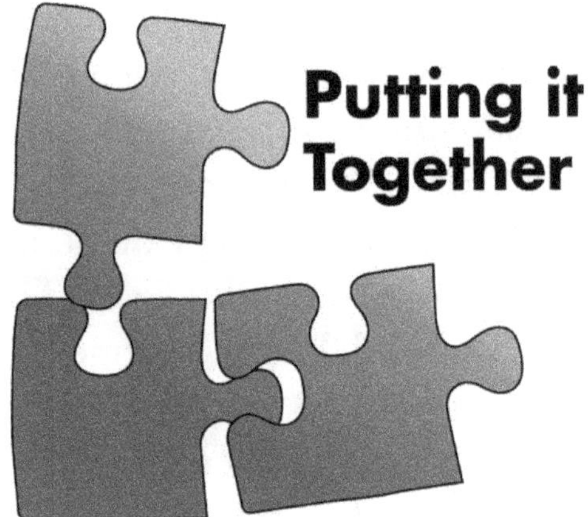
Putting it
Together

Songs are important—they are cultural. *It is an integral part of human experience. No matter how much of the thought process a loved one loses, music resides in the soul.*

Is your loved one a singer? Songs are a wonderful way to keep connected. The song someone learned when they were eight will still remain with them when they are 80.

Song sets for each person is as individual as their fingerprints. Find your person's 'heart songs'. If you don't already know, try Googling to find out which songs were popular during their formative years.

Also, try putting some of their 'heart' music on a recording device such as an MP3 player. Headphones can help get the sound directly into their brain.

Story after story has been told of how music raised the level of awareness and alertness in some folks after listening to a song.

"I'm in awfully good shape
for the shape I'm in."

- Muriel Blankenship

Chapter 3

Something's Fishy

It all began when someone read an article about ranchers who routinely put goldfish in their water troughs to keep the algae down. Mama and Daddy were still living in their little cottage on a few acres at the time. They had two water troughs in their cow pasture. We thought it would be fun to give it a try, so we went to the pet store and picked up some gold fish.

Mama really took to the idea. She seemed to enjoy watching the little fish swim about, so much so that we actually moved one of the troughs from the pasture to the yard and set it in a shady spot under a tree. We placed a few chairs next to it so Mama could sit comfortably and watch the fish swim.

Unfortunately, the little fish wouldn't eat the algae, and we didn't want them to starve, so we bought some fish food.

We also bought some snails, hoping they would eat the algae. The snails weren't that great at it either, so about once a week my husband and I would end up cleaning all the algae from the sides of the trough.

One day, as we were watching the fish—by then Mama had given them names—we noticed they were getting rather round.

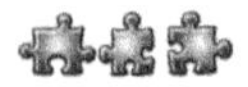

"We thought it would be fun to give it a try, so we went to the pet store and picked up some gold fish."

We asked Mama how often she fed the fish, and she said "*about once a day.*" Since the fish food was disappearing at an alarmingly rapid rate, we suggested she only give them a little bit at a time. Daddy overheard us and said he thought she was feeding them more often, but Mama assured him that it was only once a day.

Right then, she looked into the trough and said, "*See, they need food. I'll feed them right now.*"

She had fed them when we first arrived. We realized then that she was forgetting they had been fed. If she didn't see any food floating on the water, she would feed them. Again. After that we hid the fish food.

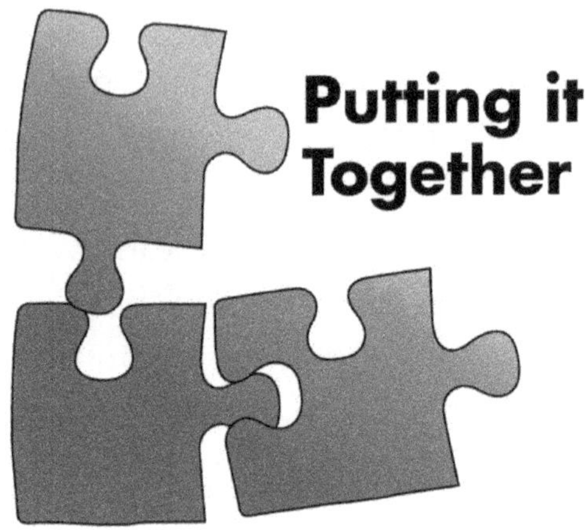
Putting it
Together

Everyone needs to have a purpose. *If it is at all possible, find a project for your loved one. Feeding fish that are lovely to watch is a good example. In hindsight, we would have metered out the amount of fish food available each day instead of hiding it: then Mama could have continued feeding them.*

Fishing is also an idea, if your loved one would rather catch them than feed them. For fishermen, this could include digging for worms.

Inside projects could include finding mobiles or music boxes that need winding. The instant reward of music or movement can be a source of genuine pleasure. If your loved one enjoys gardening, a time of weeding or watering plants could also be a fitting part of the puzzle.

"You cannot do a kindness too soon, for you never know how soon it will be too late."

- Ralph Waldo Emerson

Chapter 4

Looping Back Around

There was a season of time in Mama's early stages of dementia that she talked in what we referred to as her '*loop*'. This was before we really understood that Mama was suffering from dementia. Her 'loop' was any statement she grabbed onto and, unbeknownst to her, would say over and over again.

Mama even had a '*tell*' that let us know that the next words out of her mouth were going to be her current 'loop' statement. She would take a quick intake of breath, hold up her forefinger and begin to make the statement as if she had just thought of it. At first it was just every so often, and she would have a variety of statements to repeat, but as time went on, it became her main topic of conversation.

For example, we would be talking about the fish, and she would say: (*quick intake of breath and forefinger up*) "The roses are blooming nicely; you should take some home with you."

"Thank you, Mama," I would usually reply. "Aren't the goldfish are looking real pretty?"

"Yes," Mama would respond, "except for the little one. He looks a bit splotchy. (*Quick intake of breath and forefinger up*) Oh, the roses are blooming nicely; you should take some home with you."

"Okay, I'd like that. Are you getting hungry yet Mama?"

"No, I'm fine." (*Quick intake of breath and forefinger up*) "Oh, the roses are blooming nicely; you should take some home with you."

"Mama even had a 'tell' that let us know that the next words out of her mouth were going to be her current 'loop' statement."

And so it would go. On a good note, we made attempts to add helpful statements to her '*loop*' by saying such things as: "It's not a good idea to walk on the highway; keeping to the back roads on your walk is safer."

Our hope was that if she latched onto our statements by adding them to her 'loop', she would stay away from the busy highway during her walks with Duke, her four-legged walking partner.

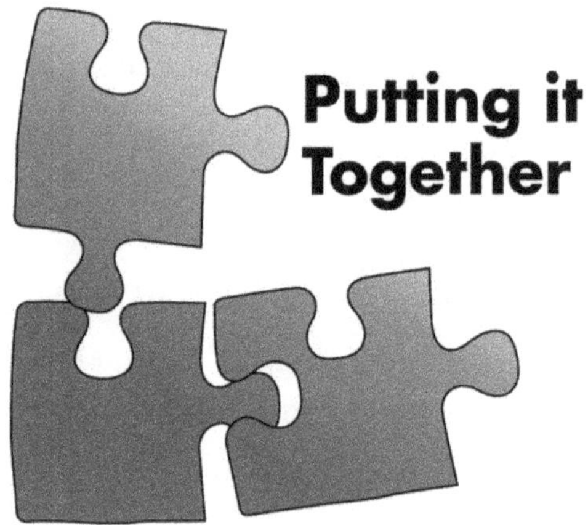
Putting it
Together

Pay attention to their words. *If you notice your loved one making repeated statements, or asking the same questions over and over again, this could be the beginnings of dementia. Keep in mind, we all have our pet stories and statements that we tend to use with greater frequency! Don't be too hasty in judging that someone has a condition.*

Every case will be different, but if it's simply an occasional occurrence bringing it up could trigger fears and frustrations. On the other hand, this could be a good time to interject positive and encouraging statements into their loop. If you do notice it happening more than occasionally, it is probably time to gently broach the subject with your loved one.

Seeking help from a medical professional whose practice includes memory care may even discover an issue that can be treated. What's more, there may be non-dementia related reasons that a person begins to repeat themselves.

"Behind every caregiver is a substantial amount of coffee!"

- AgingCare.com

Chapter 5

Coffee Story

We had a dilemma. We noticed that Daddy didn't seem to have much of an appetite and was growing quite thin, while Mama, on the other hand, was actually expanding in size due to her inability to eat sensibly.

I came up with an idea to help counter Daddy's issue: an afternoon snack. First, I would put some bread in the toaster and get a pot of coffee perking. The yummy aroma from the toasting bread and the brewing coffee would fill their little cottage with good smells, and helped perk up Daddy's senses and even stimulate his appetite a bit. In order to give him the extra calories he needed, I would add Hershey's® syrup to his coffee.

Unfortunately, that ended up causing a problem for Mama, who needed fewer calories. When she saw what was in Daddy's cup she'd want chocolate in hers as well.

The issue was solved by getting a package of paper coffee cups with lids. After brewing the coffee, I would pour a tiny bit of it into Daddy's cup, add heaps and heaps of Hershey's syrup and fill it the rest of the way up with Ensure®

Then for Mama's coffee cup, I would fill it almost all the way up with coffee and add some non-fat flavored creamer. Once I put the lid on each one, inserted straws (and marked which was which), I would hand them their special toast and coffee treats.

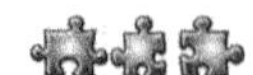

"Coffee was one of the few things we could all agree on. Well, coffee and singing."

Daddy must have known that his was mostly sweet, warm cocoa instead of coffee, but he never let on, and Mama never suspected a thing—she simply enjoyed her snack.

At this stage in their lives, Mama and Daddy were still living what they would consider 'independent lives,' meaning that they didn't always realize how needy and helpless they were becoming.

The more we stepped in, the more we discovered that there were differing opinions on some aspects of their care and living styles. However, coffee was one of the few things we could all agree on. Well, coffee and singing.

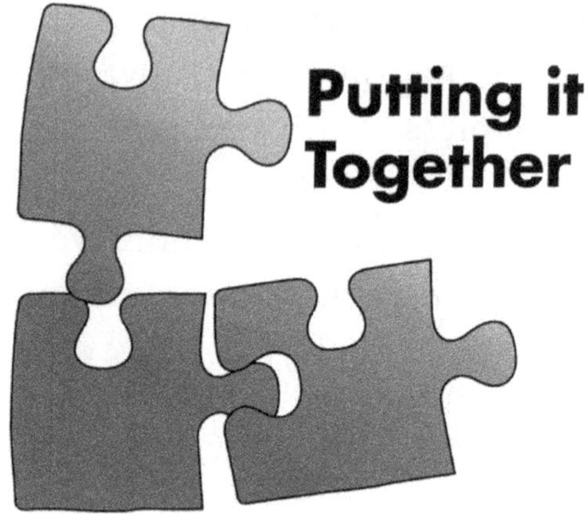
Putting it
Together

Diet is important. *It is a major factor in your loved one's daily care. Be aware of their nutritional needs – their concerns, likes and dislikes. Also, if there are any medical conditions such as high cholesterol or diabetes, explore recipes that can fit nicely into their dietary requirements as well as be enjoyed.*

It may take a bit of trial and error, but try to find creative ways to stimulate appetite or satisfy cravings based on what your loved one needs. Be circumspect. Don't try to make all the food changes at one time.

Learn as much as you can about both their nutritional needs and nutrition in general. If Googling is not an option, perhaps a trip to the library might provide you with some helpful information.

"And now these three remain: faith, hope and love. But the greatest of these is love." NIV

1 Corinthians 13:13

Chapter 6

Faith and Clipboards

Mama's faith played a large part in her life. Her values were an expression of her beliefs. Mama began attending an Episcopal Church at a young age. She went through all the church classes and was baptized and confirmed. She and Daddy were also married in an Episcopal Church.

Mama's faith wasn't an institution; it was her life. Her love for God has been evident throughout her lifetime. Mama naturally wove church activities into our family life and culture during our upbringing.

To this day I carry vivid memories of the comforting smell of hymnals in wooden pews and the distinctive aroma of the Communion elements. Mama attended church as long as she was able to. After moving into the care-home, Rev. Maryly Adair from the Episcopal Church visited her there and administered communion.

Singing became an important focus during this season, an activity Mama had enjoyed for over 80 years. It was a source of joy for all of us when we realized that, while Mama's memories continued to fade, her ability to sing continued to remain strong.

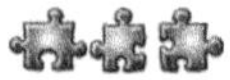

"Singing became an important focus during this season, an activity Mama had enjoyed for over 80 years."

While Daddy was still alive, we began the practice of singing hymns after 'coffee time.' At first we were limited to a couple of verses of "*Amazing Grace*" as they struggled to remember the words to favorite hymns. Since hymns have so many verses, it turned out that I also had trouble remembering all the words to all the verses—and I don't have dementia!

I Googled our favorite hymns, printed out three sets of each and snapped them onto clipboards that

Daddy happened to have (*he always had odd items lying about*) so they would stay together and always be handy. From then on, as soon as the coffee was ready, we grabbed our clipboards and commenced with singing.

Mama's favorite song was "*Amazing Grace*" and we sang every verse, including the one that repeats "*Praise God*" over and over. Daddy's favorite song was "*The Old Rugged Cross*"—we sang that one over, and over, and over. Other songs included "*What a Friend we Have in Jesus*" "*It is Well with My Soul*" and the "*Battle Hymn of the Republic*".

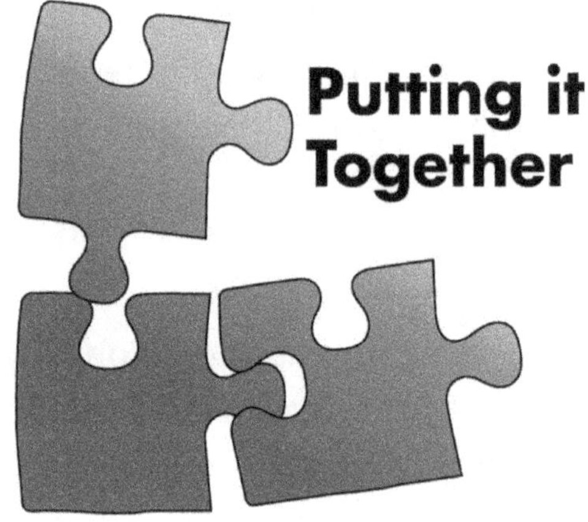
Putting it
Together

Hymns are valuable. *I believe they teach us the Gospel, our faith, and our history. Hymns tell us where we came from and where we are going. They provide a wonderful way to keep your loved one connected to his or her faith.*

If printing hymns is not an option, perhaps a local church would be willing to lend you a hymnal for a period of time.

What is your loved one's religious background? Are they a member of a church? Is church attendance still possible or not? If not, perhaps you could arrange for a pastor or priest to visit.

Reading to your loved one from the Bible or a prayer book would also be a benefit. Another idea is to get the Bible on CD or in a digital format.

I would oftentimes play the Bible on CD for Mama when I put her to bed. It seemed to make a difference—I believe the words and the sound of the voice reading were a comfort to her.

"Animals are such agreeable
friends - they ask
no questions, they pass
no criticisms."

- George Eliot

Chapter 7

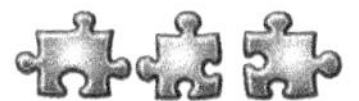

Walking with Duke

Mama and Daddy didn't own any pets, other than the fish.

Their neighbor however, owned an old gray Queensland Heeler named Duke. Duke loved Mama and Daddy so much that he bounded over to their house every morning as soon as he could get loose. We called him their virtual pet.

Duke would hang out with Mama and Daddy all day long, soaking up their love and attention (*and snacks*). It was a really great deal. They were able to enjoy a wonderfully-trained and loving dog without the responsibility of being pet owners.

Queensland Heelers are quite intelligent and capable of performing a variety of tasks, both with and for their humans, and Duke was no exception. They are also known for having a good nature and a willingness to please.

One of Duke's favorite activities was herding. If he was out in the pasture with the cows, he would herd them into little groups. He also liked to herd Mama. She and Duke would go out at least once a day for a long walk. Duke '*herded*' her up and down the country roads where they liked to walk. After about an hour, he would herd her home.

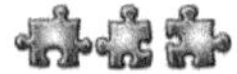

Duke loved Mama and Daddy so much that he bounded over to their house every morning as soon as he could get loose.

We never had to worry about Mama when she was out with Duke. He was a watchdog and loving companion all rolled up in one bundle of fur. He knew his job and he was very good at it. Duke was also protective of Mama and Daddy so it made us feel as if they were a bit safer with Duke around.

Interestingly enough, two weeks after Daddy's passing, and when Mama left the cottage to live with us, Duke died—probably from a broken heart.

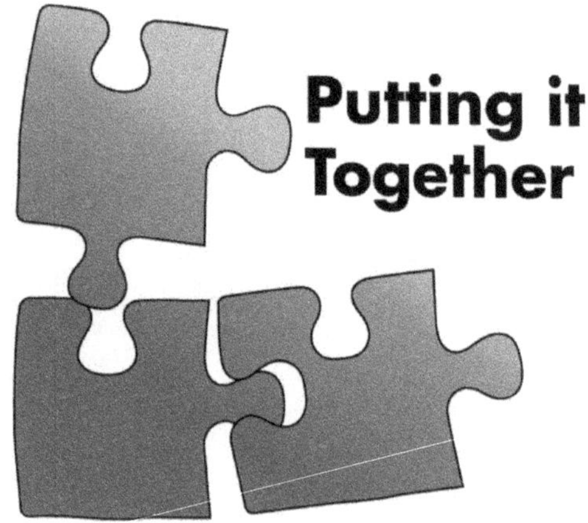
Putting it
Together

Pets are a win-win: everyone benefits. *If your loved one already has a pet, then you simply need to encourage and affirm the activities required for pet care. If not, and unless they are allergic, try to include pets into the relationship.*

If you are not sure what type of companion would be best, see if you can arrange some 'trial visits' from friends who have a pet that might be a good fit. The kind of critter doesn't matter, it's the connection that's important—a part of the exercise program.

If being a pet owner isn't a good option, consider borrowing one to bring over for a visit once in a while. Interaction with little ones could also be enjoyable. Does your loved one have grand or great grandchildren who would be able to occasionally to stop by for a visit?

Whether grandchildren, goldfish or Fifi, the act of smiling at a baby, or tending to a pet can benefit all involved.

"From home to home,
and heart to heart,
from one place to another.
The warmth and joy of
Christmas, brings us closer
to each other."

- Emily Matthews

Chapter 8

Christmas Letters

About a decade ago, I came across five or six annual Christmas letters that Mama had written when I was a little girl. I immediately sat down and read them, re-living the memories as I read along. It inspired me to begin my own practice of writing annual Christmas letters.

Mama's yearly letter writing was a practice she loved. They had a large Christmas card list and after completing the letter each year, Daddy's job was to get copies made while Mama addressed the envelopes and added a personal note to each one.

One year, early in the holiday season, Daddy mentioned that Mama needed to begin writing the Christmas letter, but she seemed stuck. So my sister Peggy helped her out by reminding her of events that had taken place over the past year—things that were noteworthy. Mama would write as Peggy mentioned things, but her paragraphs were very disconnected and sometimes repeated. Peggy helped her out by smoothing them together in a more flowing style.

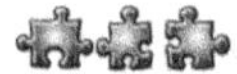

"Mama's yearly letter writing was a practice she loved.
It inspired me to begin my own practice of writing annual Christmas letters."

Unfortunately, by the next year Daddy had passed away, and Mama had even less ability to write an entire letter. Peggy and I felt it was important to connect with all who had known Daddy, but may not have heard of his passing.

We wanted to do one last letter. Peggy "interviewed" Mama regarding events over the past year and by using Mama's 'voice' in the wording, wrote the letter.

A side note:
The Christmas season is such a wonderfully-musical time. Playing Christmas music during the holidays may trigger some memories, and perhaps you will discover your loved one singing along.

Other memory triggers might come from their sense of smell. The Christmas season brings with it a whole gaggle of familiar smells. Scents range from freshly cut pine, to warm Christmas cookies as well as a host of other, unique fragrances and aromas that arise during this time of the year.

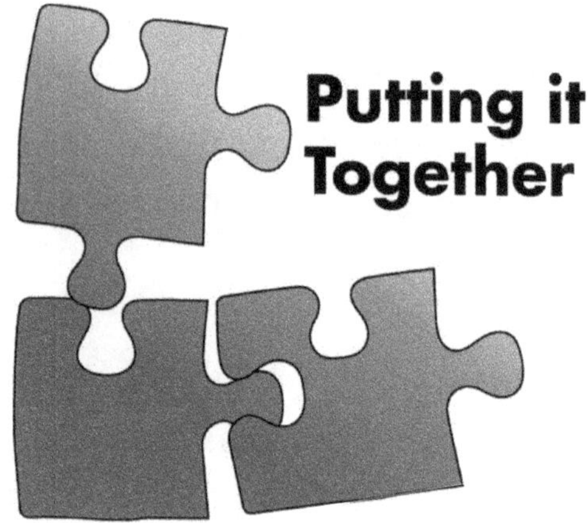
Putting it
Together

Continuity is essential to social structure. *What traditions does your loved one practice during the holiday season? Perhaps they don't write letters, but do they maintain a Christmas card list? How does she or he socially communicate and celebrate the holiday season?*

Even if sending out cards or letters is not the usual practice, your loved one may receive something in the mail from someone else. If that happens, it is best to reply to the sender with a short note explaining the health situation with its limitations, but assuring them that you will convey their holiday greeting.

If possible, take your loved one to an event such as a Christmas play or performance. However, try to avoid busy malls and noisy department stores if at all possible as that could cause additional confusion.

"The word that is heard perishes, but the letter that is written remains."

- Anonymous

Chapter 9

Notes to Mama

Daddy had just suffered a massive stroke and had been air transported to Enloe Hospital, 40 miles to the south. Mama didn't know what was happening around her. She would get confused and become quite distressed. That's when we began to write short notes to her that she could read over and over in order to help her understand what was going on.

My name is
Muriel Fay Blankenship.
My husband is Dewey
Arthur Blankenship.
I have four children, Peggy,
Senia, Arthur Paul,
and Andy Jon.
My husband is in Enloe
Hospital; we are going to go
visit him today.
It will be nice to see him.

The notes seemed to really help her—she would read them over and over, so we continued writing them on a regular basis.

Over time, the notes we wrote for her changed to reflect her current living situation, but we always began with the most familiar things: her name, the names of her children and the important point that she was being taken care of. We even included a bit of humor as my husband, Wayne, always referred to himself as "*her handsome son-in-law*". That reference always made Mama laugh!

My sister Peggy went one step further when Mama lived with her. Peggy put colorful signs outside the door of her bedroom and bathroom which helped Mama to keep her bearings and not feel so confused.

At first, she stayed primarily at Peggy's, but a time came when it made the most sense to have Mama live with us. Since Wayne and I were still working full time, we hired a caregiver to be with her during working hours.

We went through a couple of caregiver changes because we had a hard time finding someone who we felt would be "just right" for Mama, and also had enough room in their schedule to accommodate her needs.

We would write her notes each day before we went to work. Whenever she became distressed due to not knowing what was happening around her, she could read her notes and feel reassured.

A side note:
An amazing thing took place at the time of Daddy's stroke. He and Mama were alone in their little cottage when it happened, but someone called 911 and was able to give information. It is doubtful that Daddy was the one who made the call, as the stroke was massive and would have rendered him quite helpless, so somehow, with God's help, Mama was able to come out of her mental fog long enough to call for help. Sadly though, Daddy passed away on August 11, 2006.

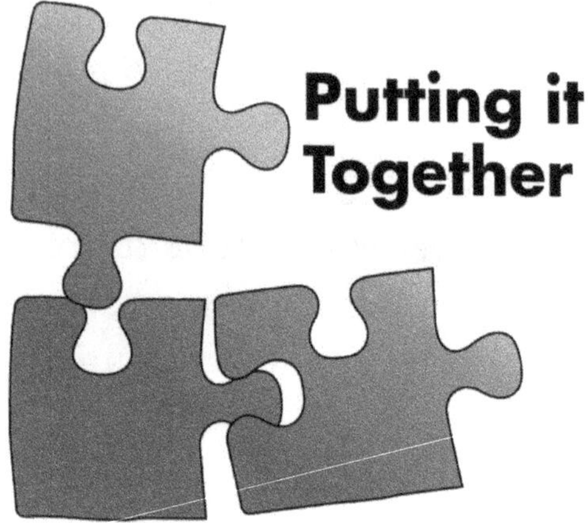
Putting it
Together

Communication is vital! *Merely talking to your loved one is not always communication. Someone suffering from a debilitating disease like dementia may have a difficult time processing the message connected with the sound from the ears to the brain. Even if words are still meaningful, they may be quickly forgotten which can lead to frustration for both parties.*

When you do have to provide the same information over and over again, it can be tempting to express annoyance, but try to have grace – remember all the times you have forgotten something. It simply happens with greater frequency to someone with a memory issue.

If your loved one is still able to read, a written message is better than a verbal one as it can be read again and again.

"Some days there won't be a song in your heart.
Sing anyway."

- Emory Austin

Chapter 10

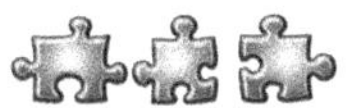

Hymnals in Binders

After Mama came to live with us, we wanted to help her continue singing hymns, so we bought a CD of twenty-five greatest hymns. I found the lyrics to each one and customized them until they matched exactly with the verses and words the choir sang on the CD.

Next, I printed out the words and placed them in a binder with a cover sheet titled "*Mama's Songs*". I actually made a few back-up copies, just in case something happened to the original.

Each evening we would put the CD on, open the binder, and Mama, Wayne and I would all sing along. We sang those twenty-five hymns over and over. Even though Mama could read, she would occasionally lose her place in the song, so I would help her by following the words with my finger. That kept us all on track and made the singing more enjoyable.

Sometimes at night, if Mama was having trouble sleeping I would put one of the CDs on in her bedroom.

I tried to set the volume loud enough for her to hear it, but soft enough so it wouldn't disturb her ability to fall asleep.

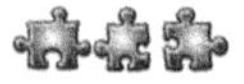

"Mama's ability to sing was one of the last pieces of herself she was able to hang on to. Even when her ability to speak was gone, she was able to sing."

Mama's ability to sing was one of the last pieces of herself she was able to hang on to. Even when her ability to speak was gone, she was able to sing. We felt very fortunate that since Mama had always been a 'singer', we knew how much she enjoyed the hymns earlier in her life and we were able to help her carry on that practice.

Songs from the past

Popular Songs of the 1920s

Who's Sorry Now - Isham Jones / Marion Harris

Singin' In The Rain - Cliff Edwards / Earl Burtnett

California, Here I Come! - Al Jolson

Me And My Shadow - Jack Smith / Nat Shilkret

Five Foot Two, Eyes Of Blue - Gene Austin

Popular Songs of the 1930s

Over The Rainbow - Judy Garland / Glenn Miller

In The Mood - Glenn Miller

Wabash Cannon Ball - Roy Acuff

Beer Barrel Polka - Will Glahe / Andrews Sisters

In A Shanty In Old Shanty Town - Ted Lewis / Ted Black

Popular Songs of the 1940s

Boogie Woogie Bugle Boy - Andrews Sisters

Sentimental Journey - Les Brown (Doris Day)

You Are My Sunshine - Jimmie Davis

This Land Is Your Land - Woody Guthrie

Chattanooga Choo Choo - Glenn Miller

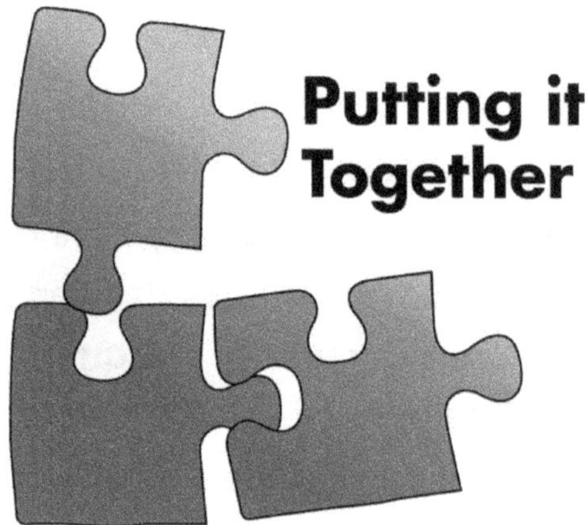
Putting it
Together

Music is a stimulus. *Look for the musical element that brings your person closest to the surface. Some like singing alone, some like watching others sing or dance on television, or even at a concert. Some would enjoy listening to music with headphones or on a CD player as they fall asleep at night.*

Try to discover what type of sensory stimulation strikes a chord with your loved one and work it into their regular routine. It might even be fun to incorporate a musical 'noise maker' such as a tambourine, drum, or rainstick.

If possible, use additional resources such as providing the words to songs or listening-assisted devices to make a better connection with the experience. Remember, our expressions speak volumes, so even if the music is not your favorite genre, a smile on your face, and perhaps even singing along, will go a long way in bringing enjoyment to all involved.

"They can't enter your reality...
you have to enter theirs."

- Peggy Whitten

Chapter 11

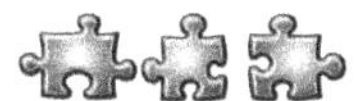

Inquiring Minds

It turns out that inquiring minds really do want to know, (Thank you, *National Enquirer*). Whenever we notice something new or different, we automatically want to know its story.

I have found that to be particularly true for those suffering from dementia. Our brains are wired with a natural need-to-know. Science has revealed that if we become aware of an object or circumstance that we can't explain, the left hemisphere of our brain will begin weaving and concocting a story to provide it with an explanation.

There was a season of time in Mama's early stages of dementia that she demonstrated this phenomenon on a daily basis. For example, if she noticed a blue cup sitting on a table in front of her, having forgotten I had just set it there, she would come up with a story about how the neighbor came by and happened to remember she liked the color blue and gave her the cup.

On an especially creative day, she might add that it had juice in it from an old family recipe. I had heard others tell me about the crazy stories their loved ones came up with and always wondered what would cause that.

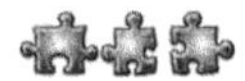

"Our brains are wired with a natural need-to-know.

Whenever we notice something new or different, we automatically want to know its story."

Once Mama's crazy stories became frequent, we realized that it was simply a way for her brain to explain the otherwise unexplainable and allow her mind to rest. At first I would try to correct her and give her the right explanation, but after realizing that she was simply trying to reconcile her world with what she was seeing, I had to resist correcting her and began admiring her level of creativity.

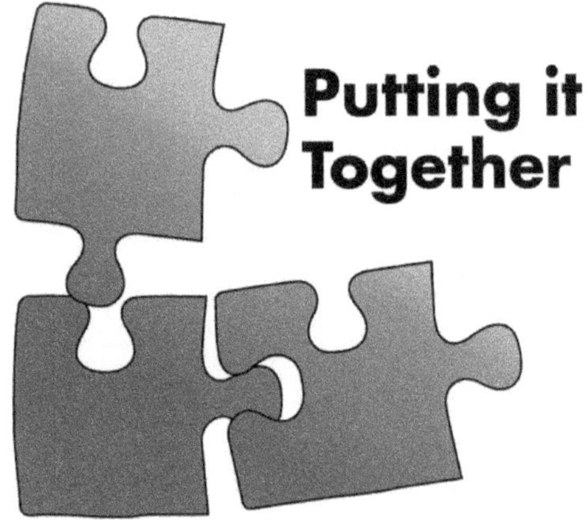
Putting it
Together

Understand what is going on. *A person's mind wants to fill in the information gaps caused by their dementia.*

There is a word for this practice: Confabulation – also known as 'honest lying'. In psychology, confabulation is a memory disturbance, defined as the production of fabricated, distorted or misinterpreted memories about oneself or the world, without the conscious intention to deceive.

Appreciate all the work and energy involved in this phenomenon. Your loved one is simply trying to keep their "boat of reality" upright and floating. As long as the story is harmless fiction, simply enjoy their imagination.

Note: A person with dementia might also be prone to falsely accusing people (including their caregiver) of things like stealing or abuse. This behavior is not only hurtful but potentially incriminating.

If that should happen, it is important to validate your loved one's feelings with empathy and express your sympathy that something is amiss. Offer to help look for the missing item with them, or try distraction therapy to break out of that loop.

"I don't remember ever forgetting anything."

- Peggy Whitten

Chapter 12

Doors and Bells

Muscle memory is what we are using when we do something without thinking about every tiny detail of the activity.

I'm using muscle memory as I type. My fingers are much better at typing than my brain is. If I had to take the time to think about each letter, and where it was on the keyboard, typing would take much longer. Driving a car is the same idea—once our hands and feet get used to their duties during driving, we can concentrate on the more important parts such as steering and avoiding accidents.

Once Mama came to live with us, we began the practice of keeping the doors leading outside locked at all times. We thought that was enough to keep Mama from going outside alone. We were under the mistaken impression that dementia would prevent her from remembering how to unlock doors.

We perform a multitude of actions using muscle memory. We're usually not aware of it on a conscious level. That is why we found Mama outside by the mailbox one day chatting with a neighbor.

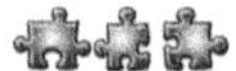

"I'm using muscle memory as I type. My fingers are much better at typing than my brain is."

It turned out that Mama's brain couldn't remember how to unlock a lock, meaning that if I asked her to show me how to unlock it, she would have to think about it and wouldn't be able to do it. But if she simply walked past a door and wanted to go outside, her finger muscles would remember how to unlock a lock, and voila! The door opened and out she went.

By the time we discovered her escape, the neighbor she was visiting with was beginning to get the idea there was something a little bit interesting going on with the nice lady who simply appeared to be out for a walk.

My husband Wayne quickly went to the ‘big box’ store and bought a new lock he could install near the top of the door where Mama would never think to look and couldn’t reach. We also hung a very large Christmas bell around the doorknob to create noise for added security.

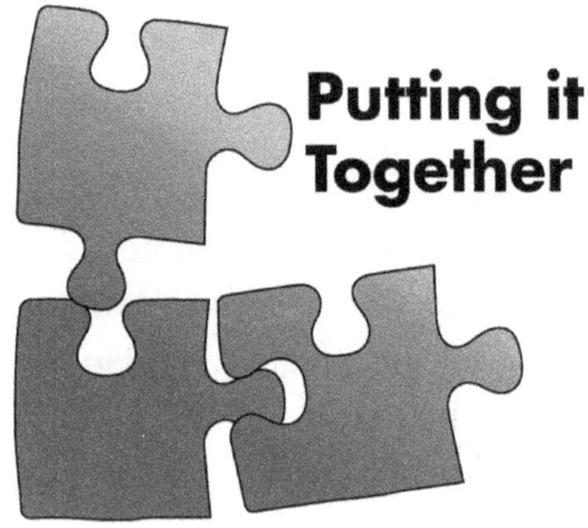
Putting it
Together

Expect the unexpected. *If your loved one was creative, versatile or showed a great level of ingenuity prior to the onset of dementia, you may find yourself with a challenge. In addition to adding bells and locks you may consider pulling knobs off stoves and ovens (if possible) and putting away sharp objects.*

A necklace or bracelet with useful information such as name and medical condition along with contact information is good for your loved one to wear just in case.

Be proactive where you can. It's the same idea as child-proofing your home and many products may work for either age group. Keeping your loved one occupied with structured activities or finding projects for their level of ability can be a helpful line of defense against the unexpected.

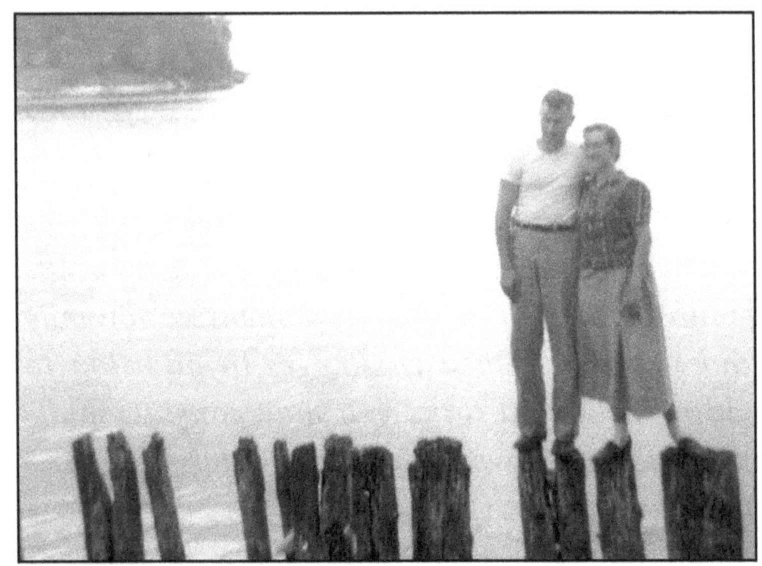

Dewey and Muriel

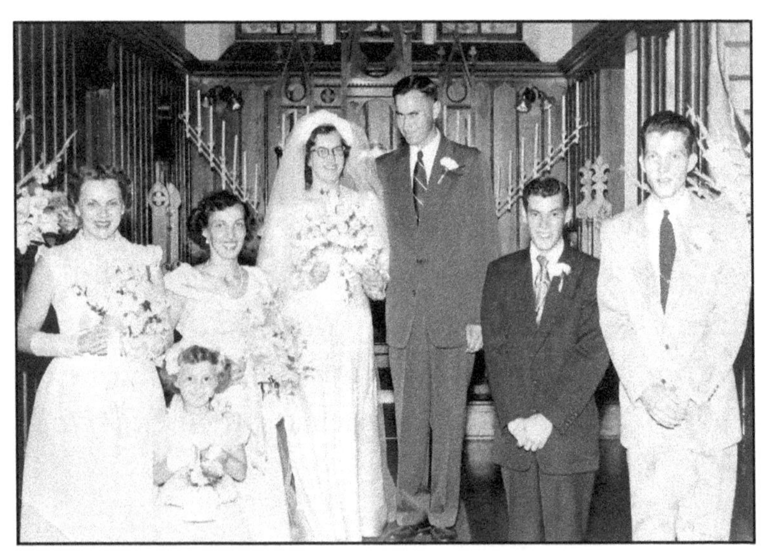

Muriel and Dewey's wedding, August 1, 1953 at Trinity Episcopal Church in Gladstone, Michigan

Travels

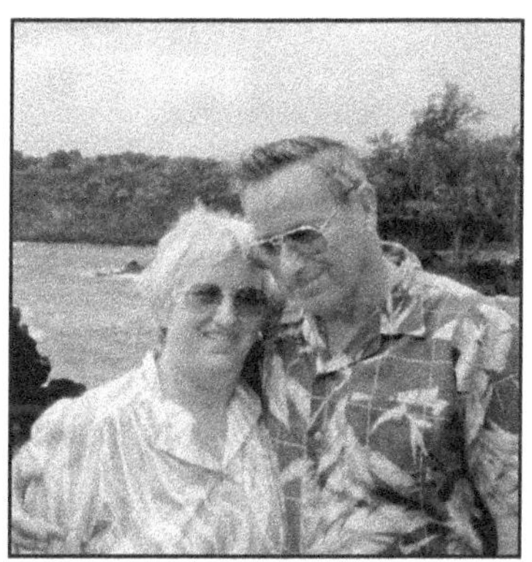

London, England

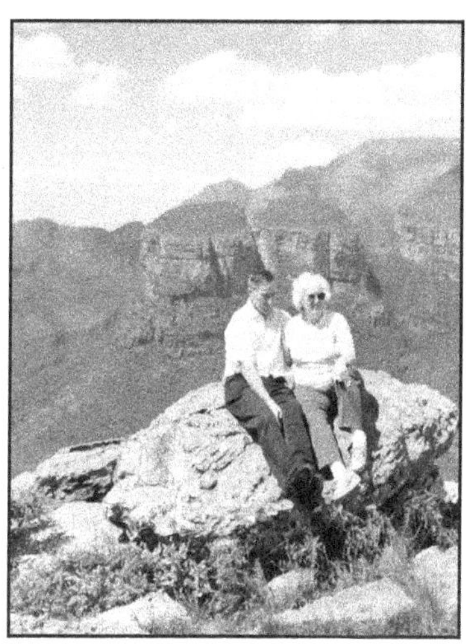

South Africa

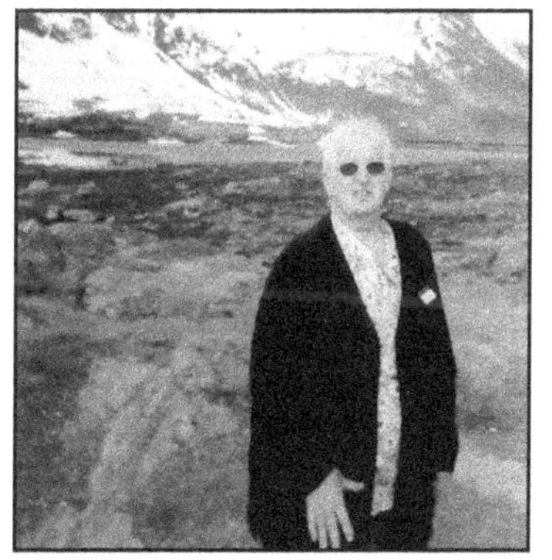

Maui, Hawaii

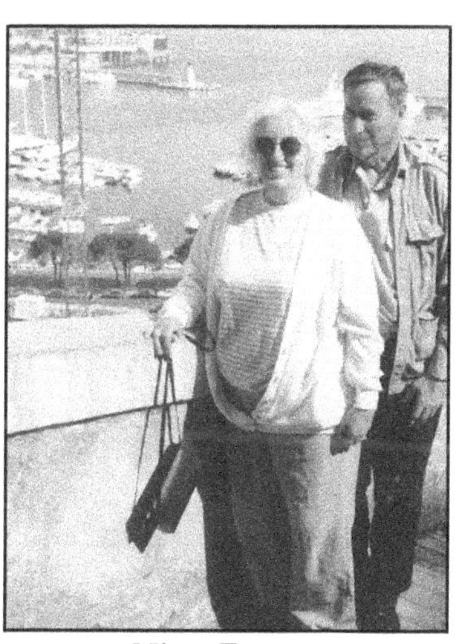

Norway

Nice, France

Family

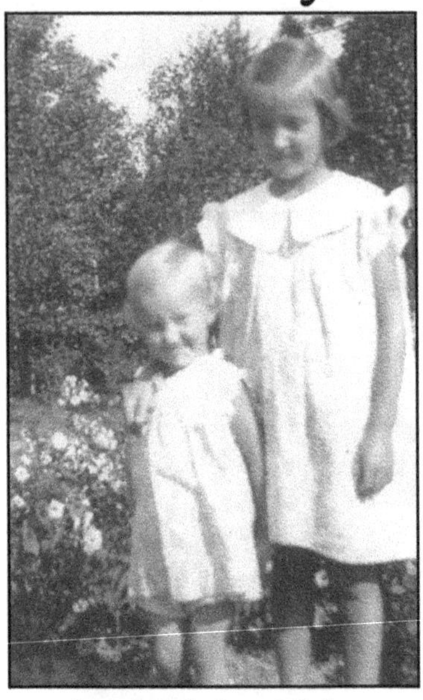

Muriel, left, with her sister, Ann Aasve

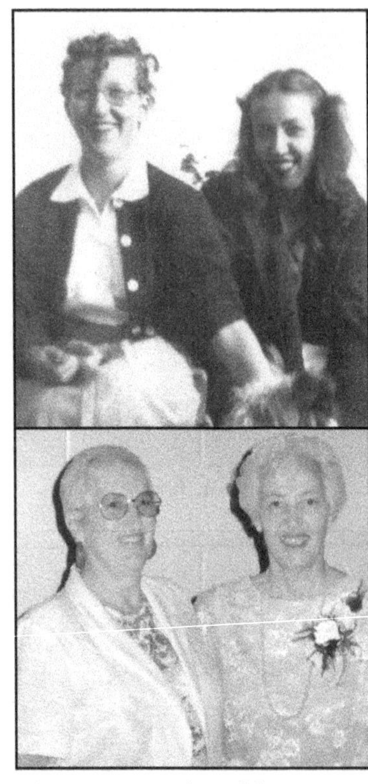

Above, Muriel and her sister as teenagers and later years.

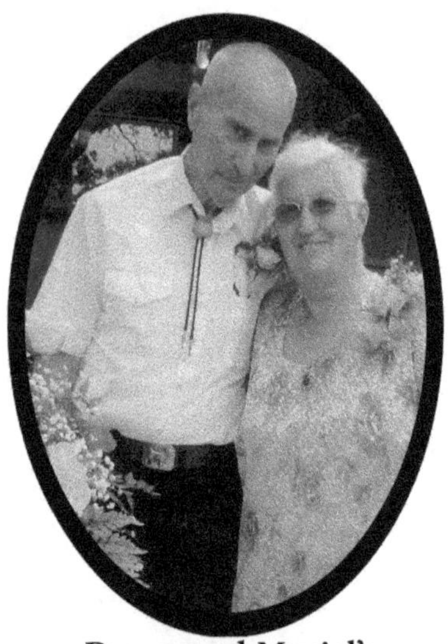

Dewey and Muriel's 50th Anniversary

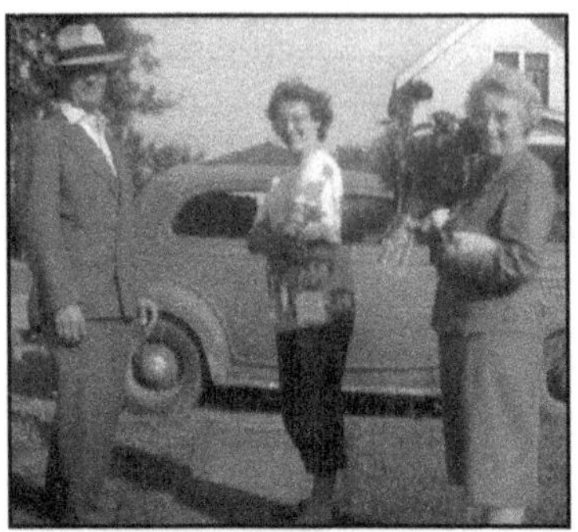

Muriel with her parents, Winfred and Senia Aasve

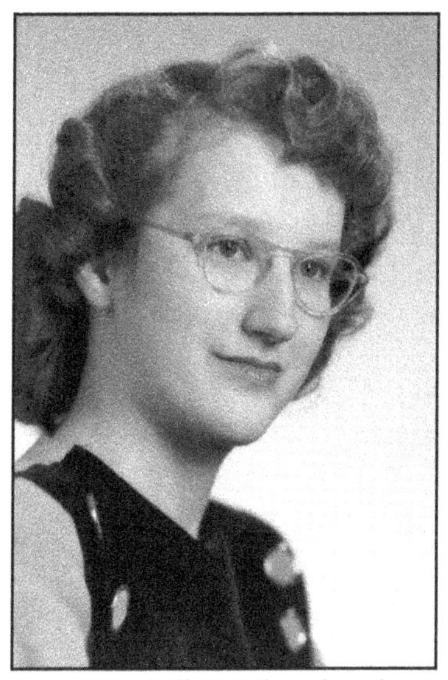
Muriel's high school senior photo

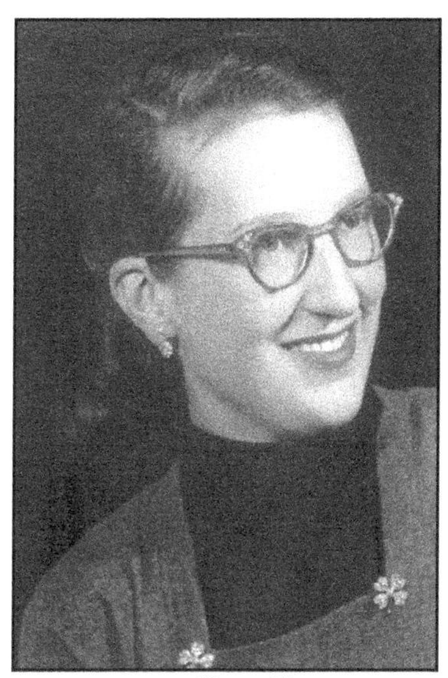
Muriel's college senior photo

Muriel loved to...

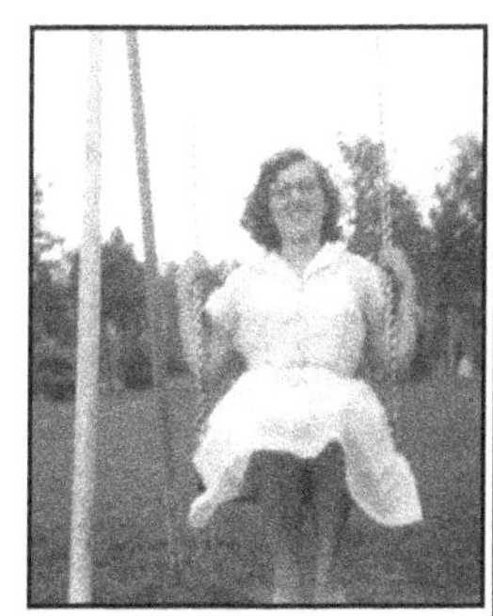
Swing

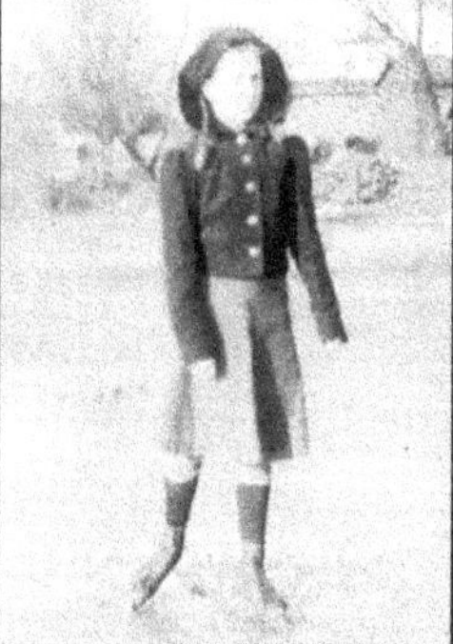
Ice Skate

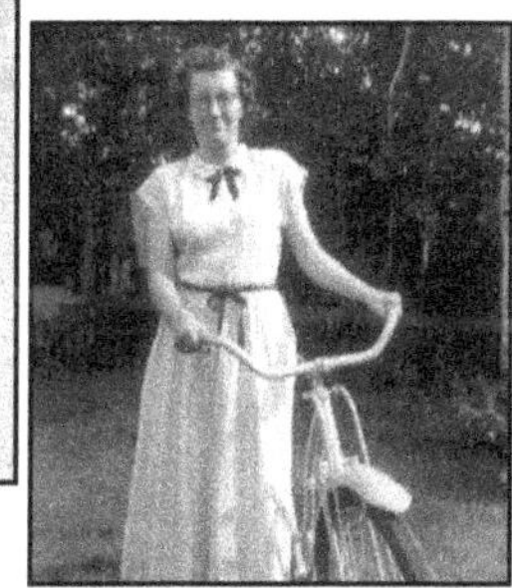
Bike

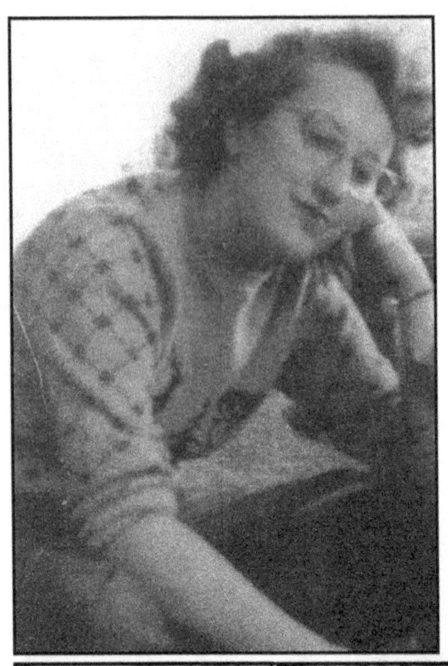

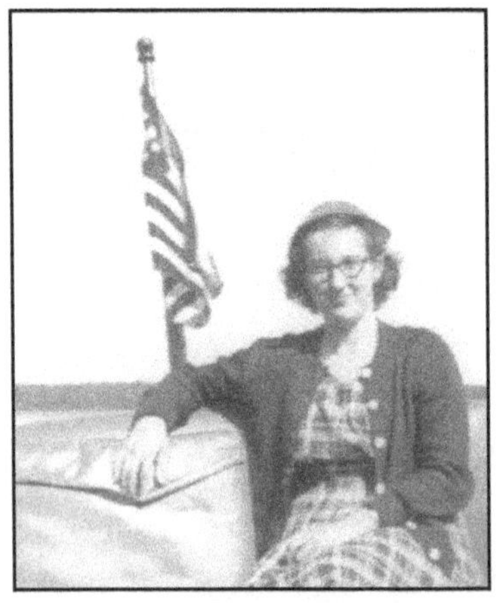

Left, dreamy Muriel
Top, focused Muriel

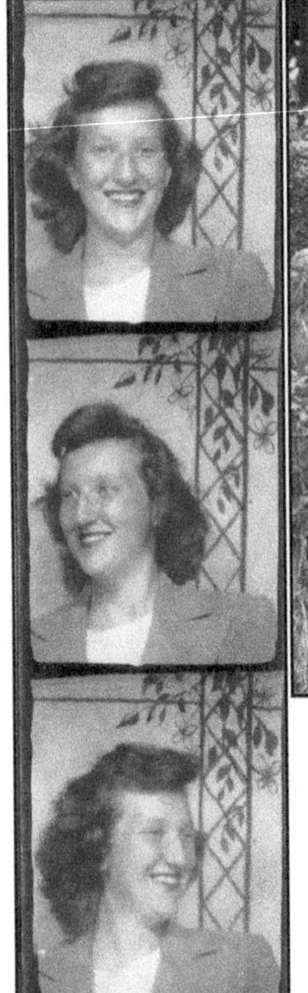

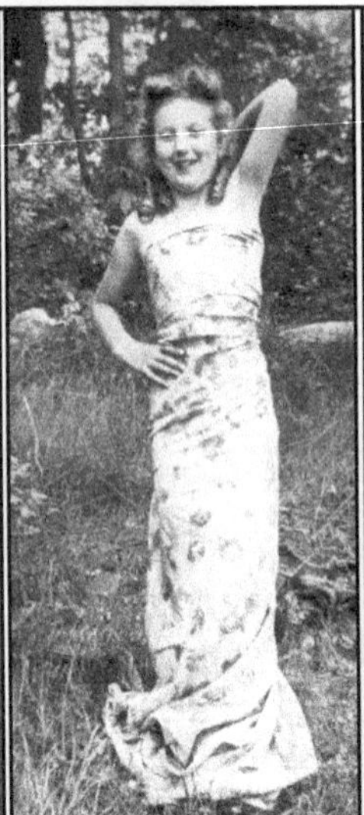

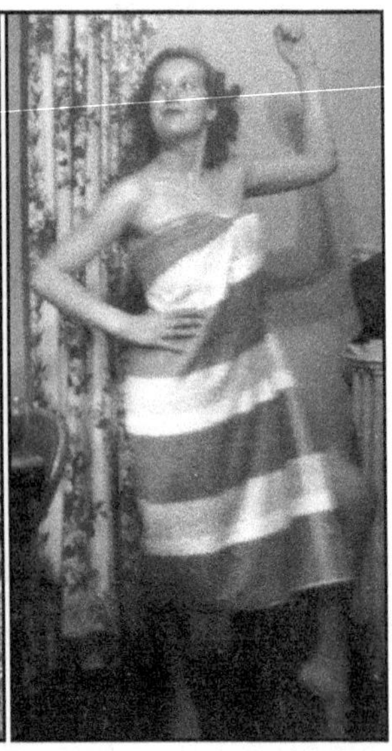

Muriel loved to be funny.
She was smart, witty
and even silly (*at times*)

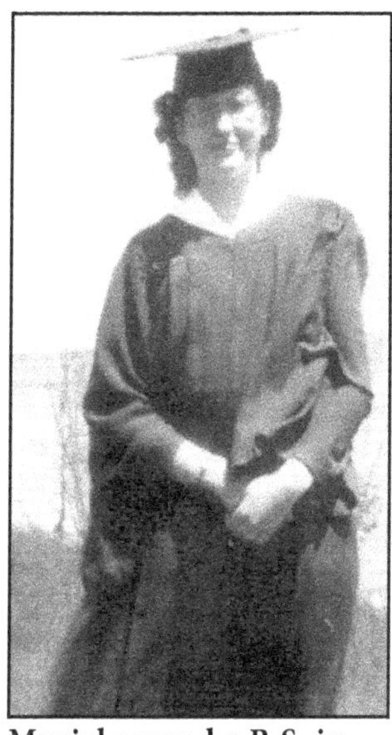

Muriel earned a B.S. in General Science (Medical Technology Major) with honor on May 11, 1953 from Michigan College of Mining and Technology (Michigan Tech)

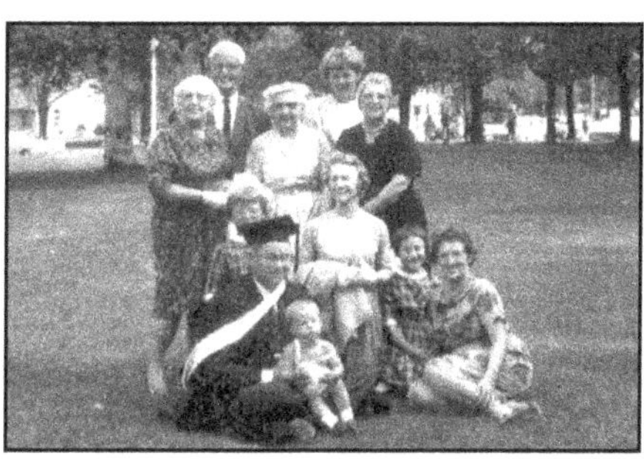

Dewey received a Master's Degree in Math and Computer Science at Northern Michigan University in 1964.

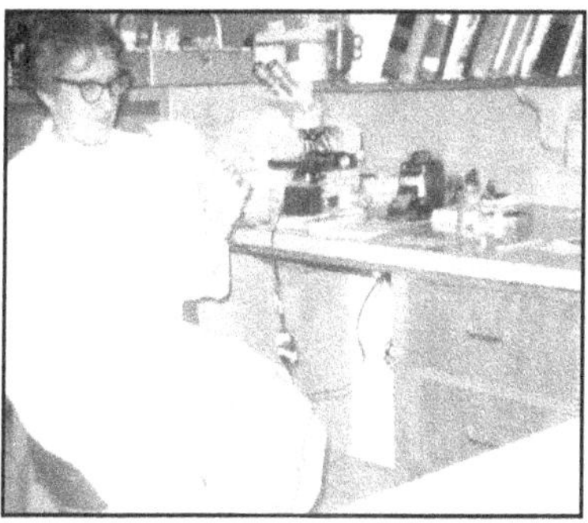

Muriel working as a laboratory scientist.

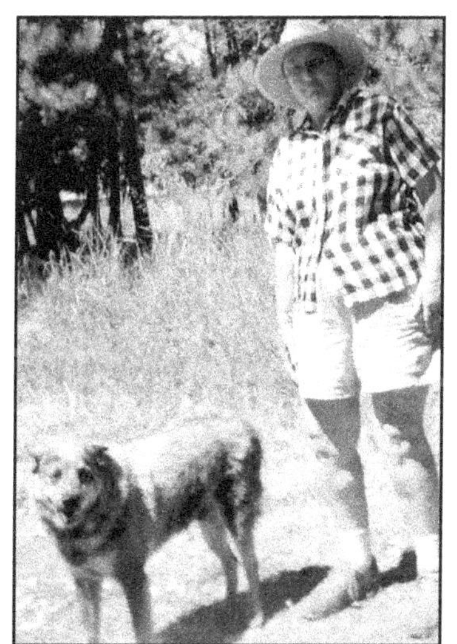

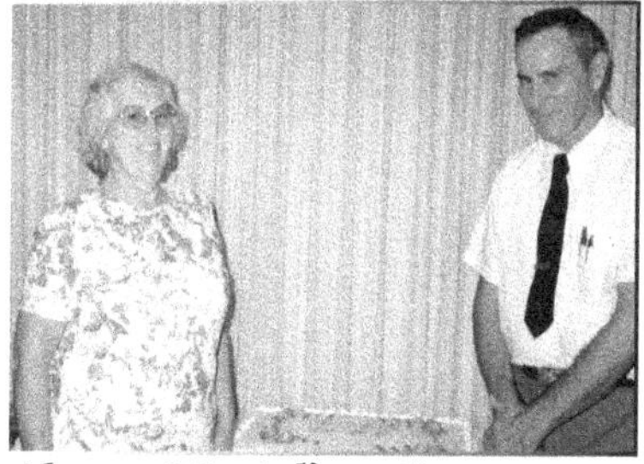

Above, Muriel's retirement party from St. Elizabeth Community Hospital

Left, Muriel and her beloved, constant walking companion, Duke

"Maturity may be a puzzle, but puzzles can be put together"

- Senia Owensby

Chapter 13

Games and Fun

Even though Mama had limited memory, she was still quite able to do things that seemed to operate mostly by muscle memory or habit. One of her favorite things to do was to fold towels. She was always very meticulous and enjoyed the activity.

We had fun watching her take satisfaction in the growing stacks of neatly folded towels. She enjoyed it so much that every so often we would even throw clean, dry towels into the dryer in order to give her more to fold.

In the same vein, if something had lint on it, she would be content to patiently pick all the lint balls off an item. She would sit for the longest time and work at the sock or shirt until it was lint-free. I must confess that there were times we didn't have any 'linty' clothes, so I would throw an old sweater in when washing towels and it would '*lint up*' nicely for Mama.

Another activity that Mama seemed to enjoy was playing two-square with me and my exercise ball. She would sit on the couch and I would stand several feet away from her. After making sure I had her attention, I would bounce the big ball to her. She'd catch it and bounce it back. It made sense to her. We could play this for as long as twenty minutes before she would grow tired or lose interest. At times, when she was really '*clicking*', I would bounce the ball slightly to the left or right of her to see if she could adjust, which she usually did quite well.

Since Mama was a woman of chemistry and science she enjoyed sorting and organizing—as long as she could sit and do it. We came up with a sorting activity for her: we put a large number of different colored beads in a bowl and set it on a wooden TV table, along with an empty ice cube tray, then sat it in front of Mama and asked her to sort out the beads by color. For a while, she would do a good job. She was able to focus and sort beads correctly into their color groups, but once she got tired, she would easily get distracted and forget what she was doing.

She did a similar sorting activity at our church, where my husband Wayne was on staff. There were a few times when we didn't have anyone to stay with Mama at home, so on those occasions, she went to work with one of us for a short period of time while we took care of whatever we needed to do. The activity Mama enjoyed at church was to sort colored papers that Pam, the church secretary, had mixed up just for her.

Another activity Mama enjoyed was the button game. To play this game, take a large button and thread kite string through two of the holes, tying it together at the end as a loop.

After that, hold each end of the loop, allowing the button to slide to the middle. Twirl the button around and around until the string is tightly wound.

When you feel some tension in the string, pull your hands gently out and then quickly back in. It might take a little practice at first. Once you get it though, the button will keep spinning and make a fun 'whirling' sound.

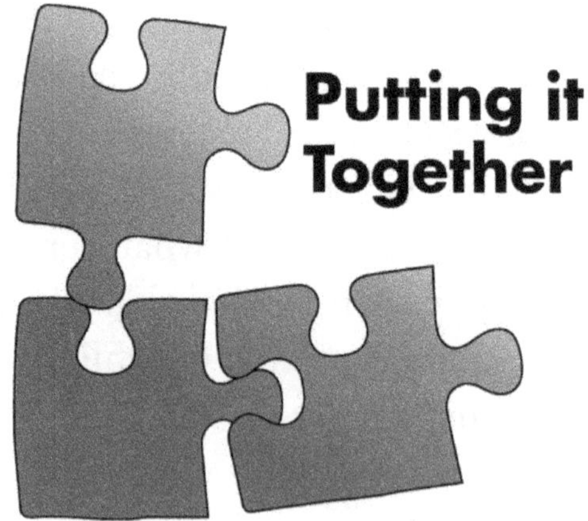
Putting it
Together

Playing is important. *Find ways to keep your loved one active and occupied. This will increase their quality of life as well as bring greater joy. Depending on the ability of your loved one, there are many options.*

Activities do not need to be structured or complicated since cognitive function is something done on many levels. Consider pastimes they enjoyed prior to the onset of dementia. For example, putting together jigsaw puzzles with slightly larger-sized pieces can make putting it together an enjoyable task.

Try to choose age-appropriate themes. Keep in mind, your loved one may have some ability impairment, and may at times act child-like, but it is important to remember that they do not view themselves the same way you see them. Remember that folks coping with dementia can tire very quickly. Time of day matters as well. Mornings may be a better time for activities when your person is more likely to have the energy for them.

"Never lose an opportunity of seeing anything beautiful, for beauty is God's handwriting."

- Ralph Waldo Emerson

Chapter 14

Birds of a Feather

Not too long after Mama came to live with us, we attended a potluck lunch to celebrate the end of a project. It was held in the dining area of a lovely home that overlooked a beautifully landscaped backyard. As we munched and chatted, I noticed a multitude of tiny yellow birds. They were crowded around what appeared to be a tube sock full of seeds attached by a hook to ornate, wrought iron poles.

I was told that the birds were goldfinches and they were eating a black thistle seed called Nyjer. The 'sock' was made of a netted fabric that allowed the birds to pull out thistle with their small, pointed bills. I found myself drawn to them as I watched them flit, fly, and even occasionally fight for position on the 'sock'. They were fun to watch. The flock was never still; they were continuously repositioning themselves and some even ate upside down.

It immediately occurred to us that Mama would love watching this. She wasn't able to bring her goldfish when she left her cottage to live with us, and though she had long since forgotten, we believed the birds would be a good replacement. The constant movement and activity that the goldfinches provided would keep her attention and provide enjoyment.

Birds are similar to fish in that all you have to do is watch them flit about. And, since the socks and seeds were easy to obtain, we stopped by the store on the way home and picked up a couple of socks and a bag of black thistle seed. We hung them on a branch of a tree not too far from our living room window.

I'm not sure how birds pass the word along, but it didn't take too long before our finch socks were sporting a dozen or so little yellow birds flitting about, jostling for position on the sock according to a pecking order known only to them. They were always in motion. It was fascinating to watch them come and go. Sometimes there would be eight or nine on the sock and two would land, and three would fly away, then one would arrive and four would leave.

We had a difficult time getting Mama to watch them at first. We would try to point them out, saying, "Hey Mama, look at the pretty birds!" But that rarely worked. If she happened to notice the birds, she would watch them for a minute or two, but they weren't near enough to her world for her to pay any attention to.

My husband brought the socks closer, hanging them both right in front of the window in a way that provided a constant show for Mama, she noticed them easily and was finally able to watch them for long periods of time.

Since Mama's dementia had progressed from the time back when she had the fish, we were pleased to see that she was able to enjoy watching the busy birds. We were happy to see her happy.

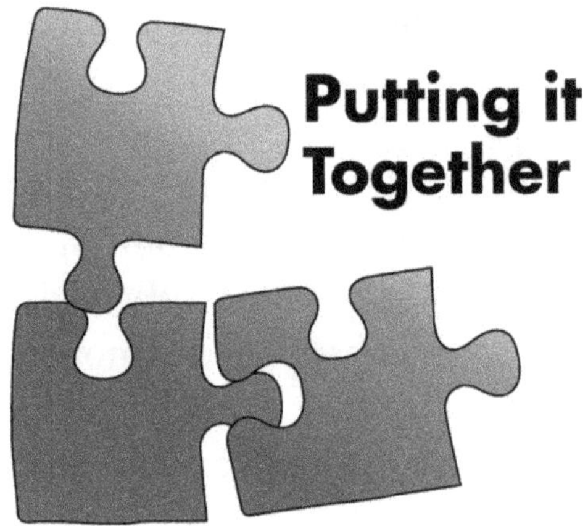
Putting it
Together

Nature offers a variety of views. *Everyday life with the things it brings can be interesting. If your loved one is inclined to bird watching, hang a bird feeder or two in close proximity to a window.*

If, on the other hand, your loved one enjoys the country life, a trip to a ranch to watch horses or cows might be pleasant for them. Or, venture out downtown to a park bench to feed pigeons. Closer to home, watching a hamster run in a wheel might just be enough to capture their interest.

Do not take for granted that every day (wild) life would be boring. Try to find a way to connect your loved one with nature. Layering additional activities can also help with the connection.

For example, tearing bread up into pieces to feed ducks at a pond can increase their involvement. If possible, perhaps a trip to the zoo would be fun. Introducing books with colorful photos of nature can add to the experience as well.

"I don't think of all the misery,
but of the
beauty that still
remains."

- Anne Frank,
"The Diary of a Young Girl"

Chapter 15

Downs and Ups

Dementia is a tough disease. It wreaks havoc on the emotions of both the loved one and those providing care. At times, there seems to be an unsettled sense of lost-ness associated with this malady. The person suffering from dementia is aware that all is not right, but does not know how to fix it. Awareness can cause frustration, agitation or even panic at times.

Before dementia, Mama always had a very quiet personality. She was a kind and gentle soul, never really a yeller or antagonistic. After dementia, there were times when sundowning caused her to become more restless and troubled.

Sundowning is a syndrome that describes a state of confusion for dementia sufferers that usually happens in the evening or even into the night. It can cause a variety of behaviors such as confusion, anxiety, and aggression or obstinacy, as well as pacing or wandering. It only happens to a small percentage of people who have dementia, but Mama was definitely in that group.

Often in the evening, our calm and quiet Mama would suddenly become agitated. She would get mad at one of us—usually me since I was the 'hands-on' person and Wayne was the 'handsome son-in-law'. We could expect a flair-up around dinnertime, sometimes before, and sometimes after.

It usually came on suddenly. We would be in the living room visiting, singing along to her hymns, or even watching one of her movies, when all of a sudden Mama wouldn't be able to recognize her surroundings. She would think she was visiting and would want to go home.

At those times, she'd stand up quite abruptly and head straight for the door. If anyone tried to intervene, Mama would get annoyed and try even harder to reach the door. This was one of the reasons it was very, very important to keep the door locked at all times.

We learned that during those events, talking to her

wouldn't do any good. "*Distraction therapy*" was the only answer. By making noise, or offering a treat, Mama's attention would be diverted and her short-term memory would quickly forget that she was heading out the door.

At some point we developed the habit of giving Mama a small glass of red wine in the evening. We wanted to be careful, so we cleared it with her doctor first. Even though Mama was never much of a drinker, she was not opposed to wine. It seemed to help her relax. We usually had only one episode per night so the remainder of the evening would typically be peaceful—perhaps the wine helped.

In spite of the sundowning episodes, we occasionally saw glimpses of Mama's former personality. She always had a sharp wit. She enjoyed making a play on words or saying something clever. Even after several years of battling dementia, there were rare times she would say something witty, and you could tell by the look of pure joy on her face at that moment that she knew what she was saying. We would rejoice with her and made sure she understood that we 'got' it.

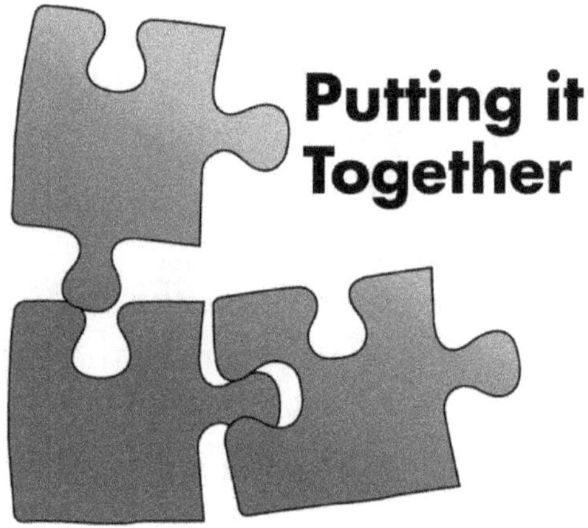
Putting it
Together

This calls for planning. *The key thing here is to be aware of the potential your loved one has for sundowning. And, as the boy scout motto goes, 'Be Prepared'.*

Keep doors locked, have noise makers handy, and think of effective distractions. Sometimes something as simple as a quick snack can make a difference.

Various types of medication can help alleviate some of the symptoms. If appropriate, even a glass of wine can be helpful for some folks. Discuss with the doctor possible treatments for these bouts.

It is very important to remember in the midst of an episode is: Do not take it personally! It is not about you - no matter what it looks like at the time. Everyone involved in the care can help remind each other that this is simply a manifestation of the disease.

"There are moments when I
wish I could roll back the clock
and take all the sadness away,
but I have the feeling
that if I did, the joy
would be gone as well"

- Nicholas Sparks, "A Walk to Remember"

Chapter 16

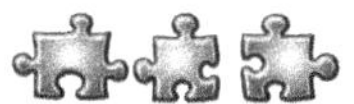

Sometimes it's Personal

Cycles are a fact of life. God talks about cycles in creation at the beginning of Genesis: "*And there was evening and morning, the first day*".

And so it goes—life moves forward: days turn into seasons, which cycle around and around each year, pulling all of creation along with it. For example, autumn marches towards winter each year, dressed in a wide array of hues. Dementia, too, can display a wide array of the colorful threads woven into the tapestry of life as we march toward our own winter. The cycle reaches completion when we realize that those who we once cared for, are now caring for us.

When Mama first came to live with us, she still had the ability to attend to most of her own personal care. She used the bathroom, washed her hands afterward, and even showered and brushed her teeth all by herself. As a precaution, we placed a waterproof mattress pad on her bed, even though she woke up (*several times*) each night when she had the need to go.

We could usually hear her get up, but one night I opened my eyes to find Mama standing next to my bed staring at me. I got up and guided her to the bathroom and waited until she was done and then helped her back to her bed.

"Throughout her decline, I encouraged her to do as much on her own as possible."

That was a wake-up call for us. We didn't want to take a chance that we might not hear Mama get up. If she was alone at night she might get lost and become confused or frightened when she wasn't able to find her way back to her bedroom. We found a large Christmas bell to hang on her door-knob so that when she pulled the bedroom door open it would jangle and make enough noise to wake us up.

When we heard her climb out of bed, we would take turns getting up with her and waiting in the hallway until she was finished with her business so we could guide her back to her room. I was taking a dance class at the time, so waiting for Mama in the hallway gave me the opportunity to practice my plies (*plee-yays*) and releves (*rehl-leh-vays).*

Mama's abilities gradually declined. She was still getting up several times each night, but it wasn't because she needed to 'go,' it was because she had already 'gone'. I would change her bedding and help her into something dry. Disposable undergarments were added to our shopping list.

Mama's showering also became a two-person project. We had already installed safety bars, shower mat, chair, and a hand-held shower head to keep her as safe as possible. Since a shower was one of the first tasks of the morning, I tried to get everything in place—her extra-large bath towel and toiletries—before waking her up, so I wouldn't need to leave her alone.

We fell into a natural rhythm of a routine: rise, toilet, shower and dress, then brush her teeth and eat breakfast. I spoke to Mama continually throughout the entire process, all the while encouraging her along, "You're doing good, Mama, we're almost done."

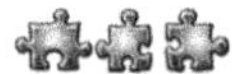

"The revelation that Mama's cycle of life was marching toward her own winter began to take its unique shape in our lives and gave my husband and me a picture of our own frailty."

Throughout her decline, I encouraged her to do as much on her own as possible. I noticed some activities were routinely done by the use of muscle memory. For example, if I told Mama to put her shoes and socks on, she would simply look at me with a blank stare. However if I put a pair of socks in her hand, she would automatically put them on. Occasionally she would even put on her shoes if they were close by—sometimes, without her socks.

The more Mama's abilities for personal care diminished, the more I found the need to intrude into her once-private activities. The revelation that Mama's cycle of life was marching toward her own winter began to take its unique shape in our lives and gave my husband and me a picture of our own frailty.

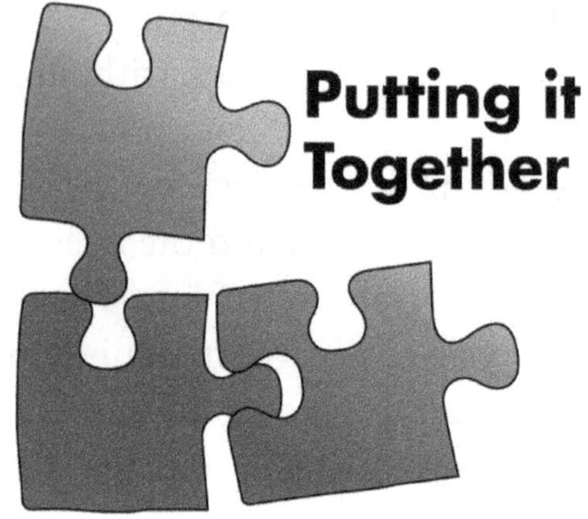
Putting it
Together

Decline happens, but don't rush it.

Remember to allow your loved one to do as much as possible on their own for as long as possible in order to sustain the momentum in their cycle of life routine.

That's our job as caregivers: to keep their personal activities as routine as possible.

Don't take unnecessary shortcuts. It would have been quicker for me to put Mama's socks and shoes on her feet every morning, but she would have entirely lost that ability much sooner along with one more piece of her own personal puzzle.

Sticking with a comfortably established routine will help your loved one maintain their abilities as long as they possibly can.

"They may forget your name, but they will never forget how you made them feel."

-Maya Angelou

Chapter 17

Scents and Sense-ability

Unfortunately, memory isn't the only thing that dementia steals—it also takes a toll on the senses, particularly the sense of smell.

Mama had always loved flowers. Her favorites were the lavender blossoms of the lovely and fragrant wisteria, one of which we had vibrantly growing on our front porch. The scent that it gave off was so powerful that even when walking by the plant, the alluring smell compelled people to stop and breathe in the wonderful aroma.

Whenever we were outside, I would point out a blossom and encourage Mama to smell the flowers. She would go through the motions and then simply give me a blank look that would cause me to try even harder to get her to smell them. I would mimic exaggerated motions of smelling the flowers and expound on how beautiful they looked and how lovely they smelled.

At that point, she would agree with me and give a polite smile; I tended to give up… at least until the next time we were on the porch. I desperately wanted for her to experience the beauty and fragrance of wisteria as she had in the past.

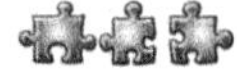

"Mama had always loved flowers. Her favorites were the lavender blossoms of the lovely and fragrant wisteria"

Along with the sense of smell, dementia also stole the companion sense of taste. Although Mama had always been very agreeable, eating whatever we gave her, we also wanted her to enjoy her meals. But without the sense of taste, we couldn't get past the 'bland barrier'. No matter what we served, she ate her food with the same expressionless manner—eating dutifully, slowly and methodically. As you can imagine, her eating method caused mealtime to take a while.

When her meals consisted of more than one type of food on her plate, she would begin by eating one thing and when it was completely consumed, she would move on to the next item, continuing around her plate until everything was gone. Last of all, she would drink her milk or coffee.

I suspect the loss of taste took away her joy of eating. It was very frustrating for my husband and me as well because we wanted her to be able to enjoy her meals – especially when we cooked her favorite foods.

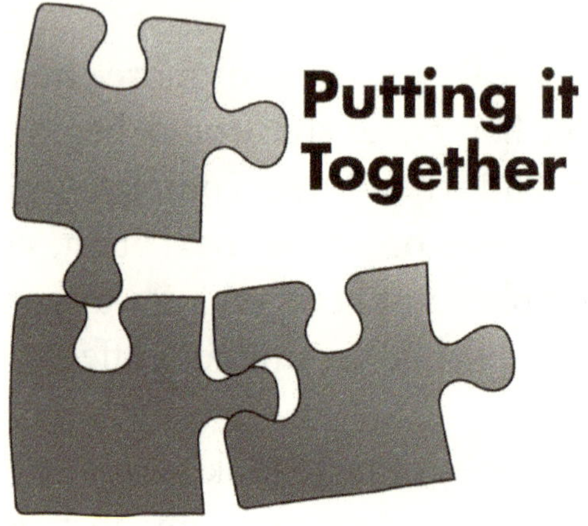
Putting it
Together

Dementia affects every person differently. *Is your loved one still able to enjoy fragrances of flowers? Is there a favorite perfume or after shave? Does the smell of freshly brewed coffee perk them up?*

There are several senses that are affected with time these are a natural part of the cycle of life. Eye sight diminishes, hearing fades. Additionally, those who suffer with dementia also tend to experience a profound loss of smell and taste.

Another sense that tends to diminish is the ability to touch and feel which could cause items to slip from their fingers.

In order to gauge how Mama's nerves were doing, I would tickle each of her feet and watch for a reaction. Since Mama had always been extremely ticklish on her feet, a lack of reaction would be very telling.

In light of the fact that Mama's senses were diminishing, we celebrated every spark of sensory joy she experienced during the course of her day.

"We're doing the best we can...
and so is Mama."

- Peggy Whitten

Chapter 18

Magazines and Movies

In spite of having a touch of glaucoma, Mama's vision remained fairly good. She had always been a reader; her love of a good mystery influenced my own reading habits.

I read all of her Agatha Christie and Rex Stout paperbacks, and she borrowed all my alphabet and cat mysteries. We also shared a love for Erle Stanley Gardner's *Perry Mason*. That passion for reading mysteries dissolved due to the dementia, along with her ability to complete her daily crossword puzzles from the newspaper.

Though her passion for reading diminished, we noticed soon after she moved in with us how much she enjoyed looking at magazines. It became one of her favorite activities, especially magazines with lots of pictures in it. Her favorites were pictures of faces. One day I happened to hand her a church directory and it became an instant hit. There were lots and lots of faces to look at. It was quite entertaining for us to watch her reactions as she browsed through page after page of all those faces.

"Though her passion for reading diminished, we noticed soon after she moved in with us how much she enjoyed looking at magazines."

One face in particular caused an amusing reaction. It was the picture of one of the older ladies with an odd expression on her face instead of a smile. Every time Mama turned to that particular page, she would gasp and point at the photo. Then she would try to emulate the expression. It was hilarious to watch. After a moment, she would simply turn the page and continue her perusal of the people.

Movies were also fun for Mama. She couldn't follow a story, but she enjoyed action and singing.

Her favorites were Sound of Music, The Good Old Summertime, and The Three Stooges. We watched them over and over and over (*and over*). She would get bored whenever the dialog lasted too long, but as soon as someone began singing, she would perk right up.

Whenever Mama was feeling rather restless, I would put one of her movies on and choose the singing scenes from the menu. In that way, we could skip all the boring talk and simply enjoy the songs.

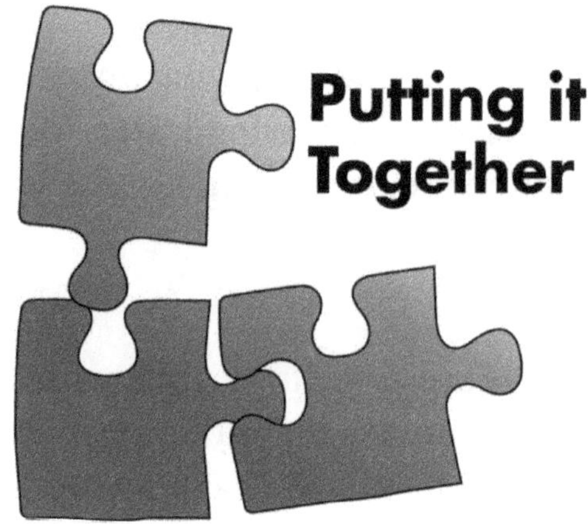
Putting it
Together

Enjoy the fun moments. *Don't take for granted or forget that your loved one has a personality. Changes in character traits can occur due to a lack of social filters. Looking for the humor in things or giving grace for inappropriate comments uttered can be a great stress reliever.*

Mama would have never pointed out the odd looking expression in the picture, but now that her veneer has grown thin, she is more spontaneous in her remarks. Remember, noticing unique features or expressions is an actual ability. For a time, it was Mama's superpower.

Along with magazines and movies, posters and artwork may be a source of visual enjoyment for your loved one as well.

"It is one of the most beautiful
compensations of life,
that no man can sincerely try
to help another without
helping himself."

- Ralph Waldo Emerson

Chapter 19

Just Asking

Mama was born in Duluth, Minnesota. The state motto on their license plate is: "Land of 10,000 Lakes," so needless to say, there was plenty of water available for swimming. Mama loved to swim.

Even after the onset of dementia, Mama loved to be in the water. We had a membership at the local wellness center that offered an indoor pool, so we took her there as often as possible. However, since we couldn't trust her to always remember how to swim, we had Mama wear floatation devices on her arms and restricted her water activity to walking back and forth in the pool.

It was good exercise for her, and she loved it. Every once in a while during a water session Mama would get into a conversation with a fellow walker. On her good days, it could take a while for the other person to realize that she was limited in her conversation skills.

After swimming, Mama and I developed a routine. We would go to the locker room to shower and to change back into street clothes. With the dementia, it was a bit of a challenge to get us both showered and dressed. I always had Mama take her shower first, and then I would wrap her up really well in towels and seat her on a bench across from the shower stalls.

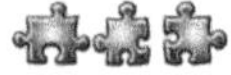

"Even after the onset of dementia, Mama loved to be in the water."

While I took my shower I could see and talk to her so that she wouldn't think I'd left her alone. I would ask her if she was warm enough. She would usually say: "Yes." I would repeat the question several times while I showered. If anyone else happened to be in the locker room and overheard me asking her the same question over and over, they might guess that I was the one with dementia.

What I was doing however, was more than simply asking a question so that she could hear my voice. I was also testing her. I could tell by how she answered if she really was warm enough, and beyond that, I could tell by her voice if she was either content or agitated.

Swimming, or any physical activity, can bring down blood sugar, so I was also checking the strength of her voice. If her response was sluggish or slurred, I knew that I had to scramble to get out and get some sugar into her system. For this reason, I carried a tube of liquid frosting with me at all times.

Mama's trips to the pool lasted until the day came when she was no longer able to walk. I believe that they added to her quality of life and general well-being.

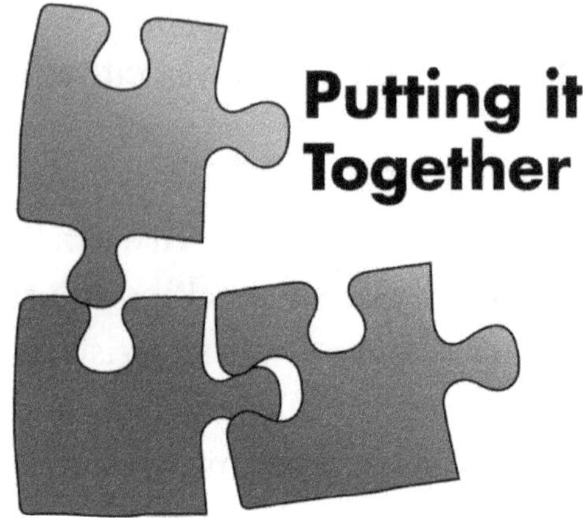
Putting it
Together

Be observant. *Your person is counting on you (whether they know it or not) to be aware of how they feel physically at all times. Someone with dementia may not be able to articulate that they have a headache or a stomach ache.*

It is especially important if your loved one has additional maladies beyond dementia such as diabetes or a heart condition. Watching expressions, observing changes in skin color or listening to voice quality are all clues as to how they are feeling at any given time.

It is a good idea to keep water handy for hydration at all times, and a source of sugar such as honey or frosting if your loved one has diabetes. Glucose pills are also available, but if Mama's blood sugar got too low, I worried that she wouldn't be able to chew them properly.

"You have six days each week for your ordinary work, but on the seventh day you must stop working, even during the seasons of plowing and harvest." NLT

- Exodus 34:21

Chapter 20

Rest and Respite

Caring for Mama was rather similar to caring for a small child. The caretaker has to be 'on' 24 hours a day, seven days a week. Needless to say, getting some form of respite once in a while is vitally important for the caretakers. When my husband and I took our respite, Mama went to a place we called her 'vacation resort'. It was a wonderful place. They had permanent residents, as well as folks who, like Mama, just came to visit for a few days at a time.

The staff was very nice, the decor was lovely, and the food was good. It wasn't a skilled nursing facility so I still had to stop in a couple of times each day to check her blood sugar levels, give her injections, and administer her medicines–but then I got to go home and get a full night's sleep!

Sadly, one night while Mama was at the 'vacation resort', we received a call that she had fallen out of bed. We met her and the staff members at the hospital. After x-rays, it was determined that Mama had broken her hip and would need surgery. The doctor did an excellent job of repairing the broken hip and she healed quite nicely.

"When my husband and I took our respite, Mama went to a place we called her 'vacation resort'. It was a wonderful place."

Once she was ready to leave the hospital, they discharged her to a skilled nursing facility close to where my husband and I both work. The plan was for her to be rehabilitated for a few weeks and then return home. Over the next few weeks we had to adjust to letting someone else care for her. We were so used to doing everything for her, it was hard to adjust.

At first we were a bit zealous in our visiting, to the

point that the management actually asked us to not come in at meal time so they could do their jobs. We agreed and cut back slightly on our visits. Over the next several weeks, it became apparent that although Mama's body was healing well from the break, her mind was not able to remember the skill of walking. We finally had to come to terms with the fact that Mama would not be coming home.

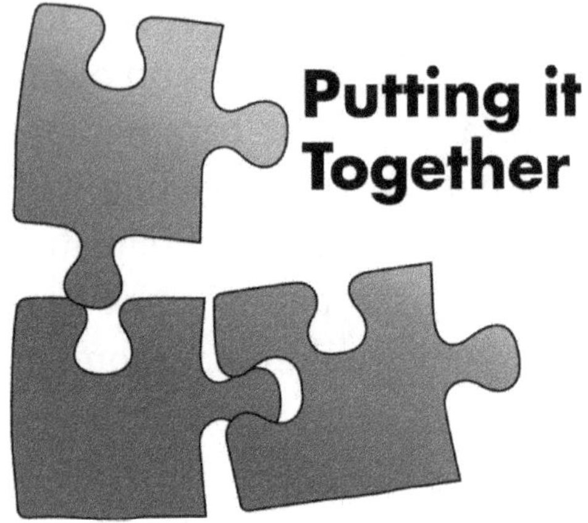
Putting it
Together

It's hard to let someone else take care of your loved one. *We know that even with the best of care and preparation, things can go awry. That said, respite is still vitally important. It is highly recommended that anyone involved in long term care try to find some way to get a bit of respite. If care-givers never take breaks, they will be at risk of making the same mistakes they are worried that someone else might make.*

If an overnight facility is not an option, perhaps a daytime senior daycare program might provide you a few hours of personal time.

There are different levels and diverse varieties of care. Find out what your options are; call your local senior center or elder care service. Are there any senior programs offered by the county or city you live in? Look into 'Meals on Wheels', or some other type of lunch service.

A call to the county social services department might be helpful also.

"Not that I have already obtained all this, or have already arrived at my goal, but I press on to take hold of that for which Christ Jesus took hold of me."

- Philippians 3:12

Chapter 21

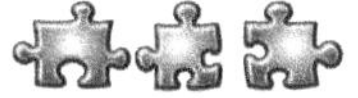

Holding On

The new care facility is great. The staff is kind and caring, and we feel grateful that Mama lives so close to us and that we can see her often. As the dementia progresses, Mama sleeps more and more. So much so that, when I arrive for a visit, she is quite often either sleeping or simply staring out into space.

I put my hand under her chin and turn her head towards me in order to make eye contact and get her attention.

I usually smile and say something like, "*Hi Mama! I've come for a visit, and I have brought you some candy.*"

Once her eyes focus on me, she will sometimes attempt a smile in response to mine. The '*candy*' is really vitamin D and calcium in the form of a caramel chewy. I always remove the wrapper before I hand it to her, otherwise she will put it in her mouth—paper and all.

Not too long after her surgery, Mama developed the practice of pressing her thumb and forefinger tightly together, as if she were holding onto something. I have to work at prying her fingers apart enough to place the piece of 'candy' between them. There is never anything in her hands, so I don't know what Mama thinks she is holding onto so tightly, and because of the dementia, she can't tell me.

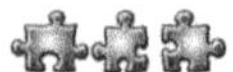

"Mama developed the practice of pressing her thumb and forefinger tightly together, as if she were holding onto something."

My husband (*who is as close to her as I am*) and I were discussing this one night. I asked what he thought she is holding on to. He thought for a moment, and then answered, "*Reality.*"

It makes sense—her world is comprised of uncertainty and total dependence on those around her. She has no ability to communicate her needs, wants, and wishes to her caregivers. She has no choice in any matter.

When we have nothing else, then we need to hold onto what we can. Mama didn't choose it, but that is the reality of her life at this point in time.

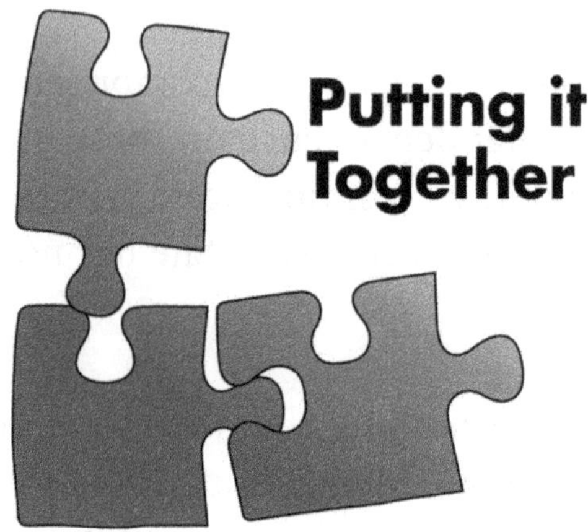
Putting it
Together

Be observant. *What is going on inside? We knew early on that Mama would practice holding on to her reality in various ways.*

Case in point: She would count her steps as she walked. At first she counted into the hundreds, but later she only got up to eight, then four. I could never tell if she was counting her steps to know how far she'd gone or how to get back.

When her reality dramatically diminished after her hip surgery, Mama would grab on to anything she could. For Mama, a grasp of reality mattered. She never stopped holding on until she reached the final stage of dementia. And, maybe that's okay, because sometimes it's okay to let go.

Even with mature-onset dementia, our loved ones are complex. It is our job to keep it simple because where she is, life shouldn't be complicated.

"When we do the best that we can, we never know what miracle is wrought in our life, or in the life of another."

-Helen Keller

Chapter 22

Rules of Engagement

If a tree falls in the forest, and no one is there to hear it, does it make any noise?

That is an age-old question. According to Wikipedia®, that question has been asked and answered in a variety of ways since the early 1700s, and it still continues to be the topic of lively debates. I don't know the answer to that question, but one thing is certain: noise or not, a person would have to be able to connect the sound heard to the tree falling in order to understand what happened.

That is not true only for folks in forests. Mama also benefits more from our time together if I follow a few simple rules of engagement.

When I am able to engage her mind during our visits, she is more likely to make a better connection to my speaking, and to the noise she is hearing. Her engagement is based on her degree of willingness to make eye contact, sing along with me, and answer my questions.

If I don't take the time to at least try, even when unsuccessful, the entire visit consists of me being a "*noisy gong, or clanging cymbal,*" as described in 1 Corinthians 13:1 in the Bible.

"Her engagement is based on her degree of willingness to make eye contact, sing along with me, and answer my questions."

The context of the verse is the need for love, and if I don't express love to my Mama by helping her try to connect the noise to my voice, then my visit with her is simply an activity for me to accomplish in order to check it off of my to-do list.

I am not always able to achieve the connection.

Sometimes she is so far lost in the world of dementia that "*all the king's horses and all the king's men*" are unable to pull her consciousness back to this world again. But we are doing the best we can… and so is Mama.

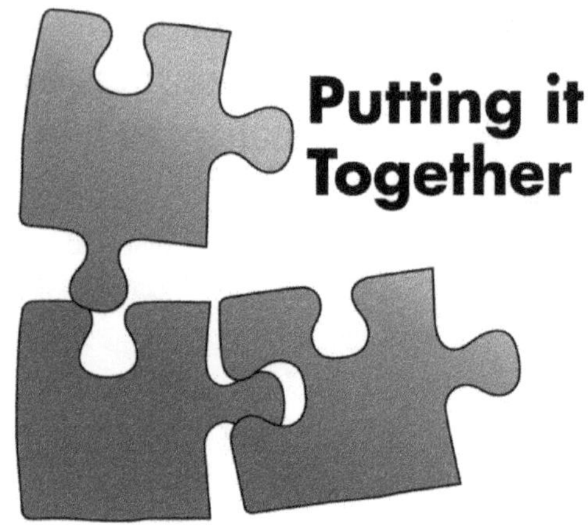
Putting it
Together

Find a way to establish a connection. *Always begin with a smile. To make a connection, there are certain things to do and to avoid. For us, establishing eye contact is our initial point of connection. Everything proceeds from there.*

If Mama is having a bad day or is too sleepy, eye contact becomes difficult. We switch gears. We use body stimulation – I put lipstick on her lips and pop a paper mint in her mouth. Holding her hand, fixing her hair up with a scarf or a barrette is often enough stimulation to cause her to react enough to bring her to the surface.

We usually visit Mama after work and it often coincides with the time of the day the workers bring juice and coffee to the residents. Mama's juice has to have a thickener added so that she won't choke, so we spoon it into her mouth. Giving her juice provides one more way we are able to connect with her.

Avoid speaking too loud (unless your person is hard of hearing). Also, try to make slow movements in order to avoid startling your loved one.

"To love a person is to learn the song in their heart and to sing it to them when they have forgotten."

- Thomas Chandler

Chapter 23

Mama's Song

"*Sing with me, Mama, sing with me!*" I begin again, "*My wild, Irish rose, the sweetest flower that grows....*" I usually place a couple of fingers under Mama's chin, and turn her face a little bit so that I can look into her eyes.

I say, "*Come on, Mama. I know this is your favorite.*" I begin again, "*My wild, Irish rose, the sweetest flower that grows....come on, Mama, I know you can do it.*" I watch as her mouth moves, almost imperceptibly. It encourages me, so my singing continues, as do my attempts to get her to join me.

Sometimes she is able to break through her dementia-induced fog long enough to sing along with me; it is an incredible thing to watch her go from barely moving her mouth to actually singing. Once she joins me, we stay with the same song, singing it over and over. Each time it usually gets a bit stronger. Thankfully, her two roommates don't seem to mind. In fact, they usually mention to me how much they enjoyed our singing afterward.

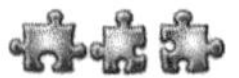

"Music is the language of the soul. It appears to enter the brain differently than words alone or other noise."

Here's some good news: I just read about a study that showed a wonderful side-benefit to music therapy. It seems that it does more than enhance the quality of life of dementia patients – it also appears to improve the mood and emotions of those caring for them.

According to this five-month study conducted in the UK, the benefit lasted well after the trial ended, measurements taken two months later showing continued improvement.

Music is the language of the soul. It appears to

enter the brain differently than words alone or other noise. To gain the most benefit from musical therapy, it is important to be engaged in the music somehow, rather than just having it play in the background.

Sadly, the time arrived. Dementia finally silenced Mama's singing. She is no longer able to sing along with me, so now I sing the songs for her.

In fact, Mama's disease has followed a predictable course. Bits and pieces of memory and ability have faded away into the misty fog that is taking over her mind. It has created such an obstacle that rare is the day when even one word is uttered. Looking back, I wish I had recorded her voice before it was too late.

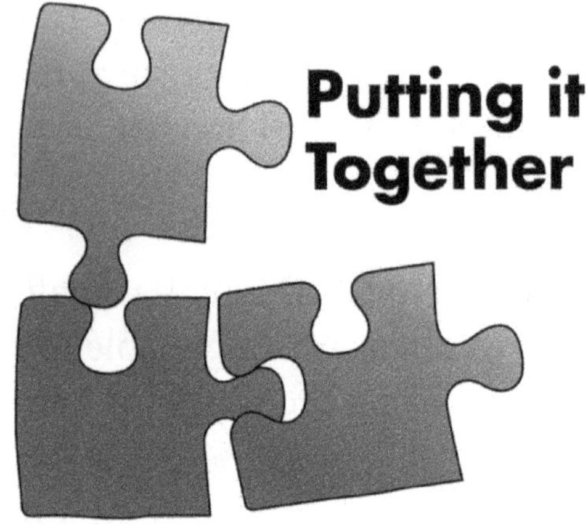
Putting it
Together

Sing, sing, sing. *Do you know your loved one's 'heart songs'? If you are caring for your parent, try singing something from your childhood—which they may have taught you because it was one of their favorites. Try a wide variety.*

In our house the songs ranged from "How Great Thou Art" to "Little Brown Jug". We know that Mama's special song is "My Wild Irish Rose," but if you can't find just the right one, perhaps you can try one song that has stood the test of time: "Happy Birthday." Everyone knows it—everyone loves it. It is likely one of the most repeated and therefore ingrained songs of our culture.

Many studies as well as our own experiences have shown that heart songs (such as "Happy Birthday") live in a different part of our brain than the place that we use for general memories.

Also, if possible, try recording your loved one singing—or speaking. Later you will be very glad you made the effort.

"There is no perfect way to take care of an elderly parent except with the most love and patience you are able to muster on that particular day."

- AgingCare.com

Chapter 24

Room With a View

Mama was a '*watcher*'. She loved watching things that moved—especially trains, cars and people, (*in that order*). Watching trains go by was an enjoyment she developed at a young age due to the fact her father was a depot agent for a railroad which was known as the **"Soo Line"**.

While Mama was a little girl her family lived on the second floor of the train depot in several cities along the rail line. She loved to tell me of a time when some of the rail yard workers used railroad ties to build a playhouse for her and her sister in the depot yard.

I can imagine that she spent hours upon hours watching trains go by.

Mama was able to pass her love for trains along to her children. While we were growing up, anytime we had to wait at a railroad crossing, Mama kept us occupied by watching for "**Soo Line**" boxcars as the trains would rumble by.

We lived in California growing up and "**Soo Line**" trains were less common there since they are owned by Canadian Pacific and run primarily in the great lakes region, so it was always a big deal for us to actually see a random Soo Line car while waiting for a train.

One day, while Mama was still living with us, we had a wonderful experience. Driving home from an outing we found ourselves waiting for a train. It happened to be a Canadian Pacific train heading north. Virtually every car on the train was a "**Soo Line**"! Needless to say, Mama and I were both thrilled. It seemed like a gift from God! And, since that day, I don't believe I've ever seen another one.

On road trips, watching cars was fun for Mama also—they came with the added attraction of license plates. She could spot an out-of-state license plate from a long way off.

Mama also loved watching people in airports, lobbies, and especially in her later years, she enjoyed waiting in the car while Daddy ran into the store for groceries. She liked walking, but her knees hurt her when she changed positions such as standing up after sitting for any length of time. It worked out fine for Daddy since she was never much of a shopper. Watching folks in a parking lot was much more satisfying for her.

When the time came for Mama to be transferred to the skilled nursing facility to temporarily (we thought) recover from her broken hip, we were delighted to discover she was assigned a bed next to a huge window where she could watch both cars and people go by to her heart's content. After it was determined that she was going to stay there permanently, she was transferred to a different room, but was again assigned to the bed next to the large picture window.

I don't know what Mama is watching now. Sometimes she is staring off into the distance and I like to think that perhaps her disconnection here on earth has given her a better view of heaven.

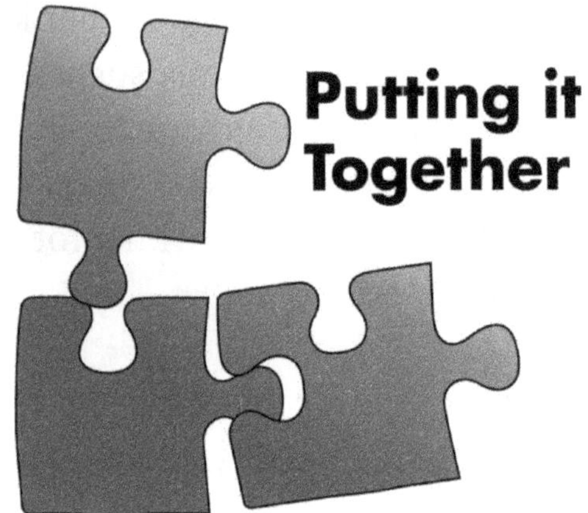
Putting it
Together

Is your loved-one a watcher? *A doer? An artist? Or perhaps something in-between. How would you characterize your person? Clues can be found in what you remember of who they were and what they did when they were vital and active.*

If you do not know, ask a family member if there were any hobbies or activities that they remember. Knowing just a few things about loved ones can offer some insight.

What is your person like now? Do they have a propensity for anything in particular? A gentleman who lives at the same care-home as Mama is a natural greeter. He sits at the front entryway greeting folks as they come and go.

How does your loved one interact with others? Try to watch them in group settings. Note what interests them. What triggers interaction? Observe what your loved one does naturally and try to provide opportunities through the things you discover.

"Endings are better than beginnings, "

- Ecclesiastes 7:8

Chapter 25

And in the End

Mama is nearing the end of her earthly journey. Her ability to chew food is now gone and her capacity for swallowing has diminished. Her sustenance comes in the form of thick liquids and liquidized foods.

In spite of her limitations, I happily discovered one day that I could still give her a treat: a minty breath strip that comes in the form of a tiny square sheet designed to dissolve instantly on the tongue. It even kills bacteria. Although it has a strong flavor, it seems to be just right because her senses are dulled from the dementia. Since it melts as soon as I put it in her mouth, I never have to worry about her choking on it. It makes me feel as if I can still do something for her.

At times I will notice her staring into space as though she is viewing something beyond the physical. I would love to know what she is seeing, but since she is incapable of telling me, I'll have to wait until I meet up with her in heaven. In spite of her inability to communicate, I believe she is still aware of her surroundings on some level.

The only form of communication she has left is through her eyes, which usually radiate quiet acceptance of her lot. That's consistent with the Mama I've always known: a woman of quiet strength, never a complainer or given to gossip.

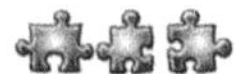

"At times I will notice her staring into space as though she is viewing something beyond the physical."

She accepted everyone and did all that she could to make those in her world feel as welcomed as possible. I'm reminded of a response Mama used to give to folks, no matter what health issue or struggle was going on with her. When someone asked how she was, she'd reply: "*I'm in awfully good shape for the shape I'm in."*

There are times now when her expression is troubled, and my only recourse at those times is to pray or sing.

Now that she can no longer sing along with me, I sing the songs for her. I go down the list, but lately, I've been focusing on the ones that remind her of the love of God and His faithfulness.
I try to remember songs from my childhood at the Episcopal Church like the "Doxology". I know she's hearing—that she's aware— because her eyes speak to me by filling with tears.

If Mama still had the ability to speak, I have no doubt that she would say, ***"I'm in awfully good shape for the shape I'm in."***

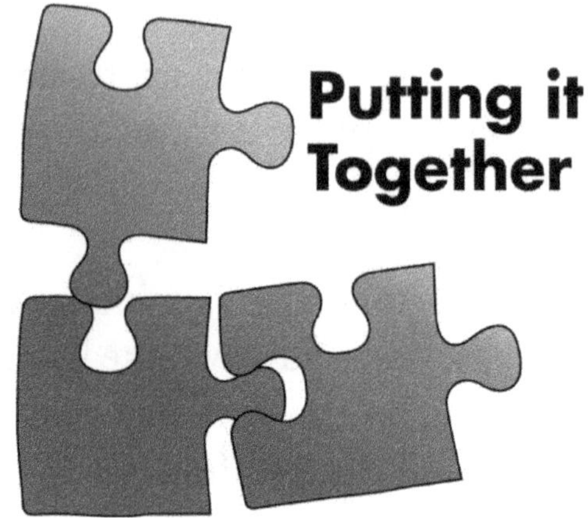
Putting it
Together

Don't miss one single moment. *Take advantage of every chance you have to visit. Try to find the joy where you can. Even on days when you are exhausted and wonder how you can go on, remind yourself of the fact that your loved one is in there somewhere, hearing, seeing, and feeling. Sing to them and pray for them. Sometimes the sound of a voice may be all you can give.*

Endeavor to speak in an animated voice as though your loved one will answer. Talk about your day, your hopes, and your dreams. Remember to smile; even make silly faces to see if you can elicit a reaction. Run through the entire gambit of every happy, funny and silly face you can—you'll be amazed—even if it doesn't do anything for your loved-one, your own mood and spirits will lift!

"The Lord Bless you, and keep
you; the Lord make His face
shine on you; and be gracious
to you; the Lord lift up His
countenance on you;
and give you peace."

- Numbers 6:24-26

Chapter 26

Blessings

One Sunday afternoon, early in 2001, a family discussion took place at my sister Peggy's house. It was regarding Mama and Daddy, about their health issues and how long they had been married. We did the math and figured out that their next anniversary would be number 48.

We wanted to do something special for them, and at the time we weren't sure if it would be a good idea to wait until their 50th anniversary came around. We decided to hold a "Blessing Party". The best description of a "Blessing Party" is a get-together where the honoree is showered with blessings that speak of the positive impact that he or she has had on the lives of those who attend—then we all eat cake.

We set about making plans for the party and thought it would be fun to make it a surprise. It was to be held at Peggy's house, and we needed to find out when would be the best day for everyone.

We contacted one brother who lived in Stockton, California, at the time. He had a difficult work schedule, so we planned the event based on whatever day would work best for him. Another brother was unable to travel at the time and couldn't get home, so we asked him to write a letter that we could read to Mama and Daddy at the party.

We decided to ask everyone to write a favorite memory they had of them so that we could put together a scrap book for the occasion. We named it the ***"Blessing Book"*** and below the title Peggy added a blessing found in the Bible, Numbers 6:24-26:

"The Lord Bless you, and keep you; the Lord make His face shine on you; and be gracious to you; the Lord lift up His countenance on you; and give you peace."

The plans were simple: eat a light supper, then surprise them with each person reading what they wrote, and then eat cake.

We added one final element to the whole thing—something that would make it really speak to Mama and Daddy about how special they were: "Soundies". It occurred to us that if we could re-create one particular activity from our childhood it would be to make popcorn and show some of the old "Soundies" movies we watched regularly for years. There were, however, a few challenges to overcome:

1.We needed to obtain a projector and screen
2.We needed to locate the movies in order to be able to show them.

While visiting Mama and Daddy one day, we brought up the topic of the movies and nonchalantly asked Daddy if he happened to know where they were. Amazingly enough, he found a box of them! He did have the movies, but he didn't have a working projector or screen. Not to be deterred, I placed an ad in the newspaper that said: "*16mm projector needed. Will borrow, rent or buy....*" I gave my phone number and waited.

We received a response rather quickly. It was from someone who wanted to simply give us the projector (and screen!), so we agreed to meet him in the parking lot at Raley's Shopping Center. He gave us a **"Bell and Howell"** projector that looked brand new, as well as a beautiful screen. What a gift!

Everything was coming together. The movie part was set, the dinner (and cake) part was set, and our brother Arthur found a Saturday in March that worked for him, so the date was set. The final tasks were to invite the guests and to try to get everyone to write and send us their blessing contribution for the scrap book.

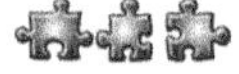

"The plans were simple: a light supper, then surprise them with each person reading what they wrote, and then eat cake."

The big day arrived. As far as Mama and Daddy knew, it was simply a family dinner with a few extra friends. We all gathered at Peggy's. After dinner, we explained to them what the real reason behind this gathering was. Then we presented them the scrapbook (*and cake*).

Each person who was present read out loud what they had written in the book. Since our brother Andrew could not attend, someone read his blessing to them as well, which included how much he wished he could be with them on their big day.

While Mama and Daddy were still reeling from the wonderful shock of the blessings, we began to set up the screen and projector. My husband Wayne pulled a movie tin from the box and threaded it through the machine. Once everything was set, we hit the lights, flipped the switch, and sat back to enjoy the movies. To our happy astonishment, the movie tin contained the '*Irish*' songs—our family's favorites.

At that moment, it occurred to us how much God's hand was upon this entire event. Not only did everything go as planned, not only did we get the projector and screen at no cost, not only did we locate the movies, but we were also so focused on the Blessing Party that it never occurred to us that it was March 17, 2001 - Saint Patrick's Day!

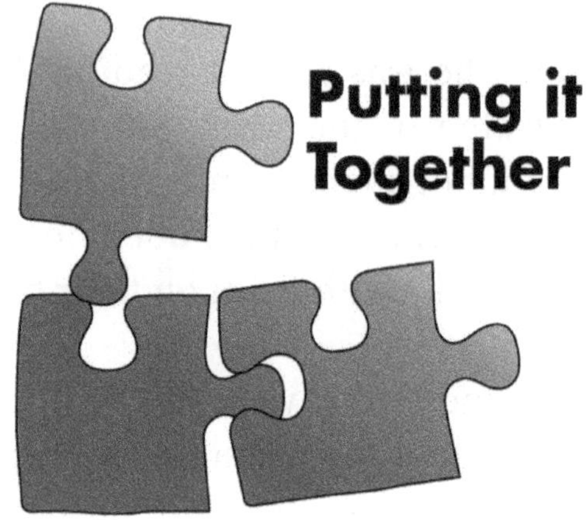
Putting it
Together

Blessings benefit everyone. *If you have not done so already, let this account encourage you to hold a Blessing Party for your loved one. It can happen no matter what stage in their dementia journey they happen to be in.*

Whether it's elaborate or simple, whether they are able to engage or to simply be present, the elements of love, attention, and wonderful words will work together and become a blessing to both you and them.

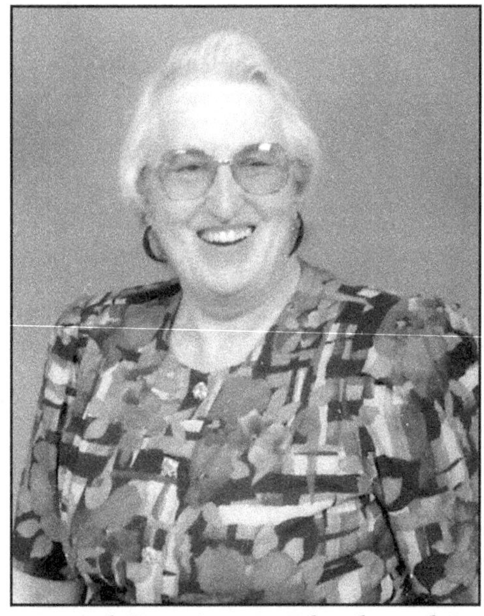

Muriel Fay Aasve Blankenship

Biography of

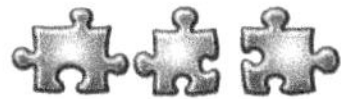

Muriel Fay Aasve Blankenship

Muriel Fay Aasve was born on February 17, 1931, in Duluth, Minnesota; she was the second child of Winfred (*Win*) and Senia Aasve. Her sister, Ann, was five years old when she was born. Win worked for the **"Soo Line"** Railroad Company as a depot agent. They moved to Thief River Falls, MN for a brief period of time and then back to Park Point (*Minnesota Point*), MN. When Muriel was in junior high school, Win was transferred to Gladstone, Michigan.

Muriel graduated from high school in Gladstone and went on to attend Michigan College of Mining and Technology (*Michigan Tech*), where she earned a B.S. in General Science (*Medical Technology Major*) with honor on May 11, 1953.

Following her graduation, she moved to Flint, MI for an internship as a Medical Technologist, (*now called a Laboratory Scientist*) at the Flint Medical Laboratory. While there, she enjoyed attending the dances held at a local dance hall. One night she met and danced the entire evening with a dashing young man named Dewey Arthur Blankenship. When the dancing was over, Dewey left with a cute blond that he had apparently come with. Muriel thought Dewey was quite the scoundrel until she learned that the cute blond was his sister-in-law—he was living with his brother and sister-in-law while attending Flint Junior College.

Dewey and Muriel were married on August 1, 1953. They moved to Hancock, Michigan, for Dewey to pursue an engineering degree at Michigan College of Mining and Technology. Their first daughter, Margaret Alice (*Peggy*) was born while they lived in Hancock. Dewey switched gears and began working for Western Electric while attending the University of Duluth, Minnesota. Western Electric wanted him to take classes in Milwaukee, Wisconsin, when their second daughter, Senia Jean was born. Shortly afterwards, they moved their little family to Pontiac, Michigan, for a job opportunity.

Returning once again to college, Dewey received a BS from Northern Michigan University in Marquette, Michigan. Following a close call on an icy road in the winter of 1960, they packed it up and moved to Fontana, California. At this time, Dewey was enrolled in a Master's program at the Northern Michigan University in Marquette, Michigan, which he could take as summer classes. So every summer, as soon as school was out, they made the trip back to Michigan, taking a variety of routes in order to visit as many national parks and places of interest as possible.

Muriel's parents, Win and Senia lived in Gladstone, Michigan, which was not too far from Marquette, so the family lived in a trailer in their backyard during their stays. The warm summer days were filled with swimming in Lake Michigan, visiting with family and eating wild blueberries and raspberries. Every Fourth of July, they traveled to Sawyer (*near Duluth, Minnesota*), where extended family gathered for a reunion at a cabin at Park Lake.

In 1962, the family moved up to Northern California to West Pittsburg (*Now **Bay Point***), where Dewey's brother and his family lived. Muriel worked as a Medical Technologist at a hospital in Martinez, California, when their third child, a son, Arthur Paul, was born.

Dewey received his Master's Degree in Math and Computer Science at Northern Michigan University in 1964. That fall, Dewey[1] was offered a teaching job in a small Northern California town called Cottonwood. They spent a year there while Muriel worked at Mercy Hospital in Redding, 15 miles to the north.

Since they didn't need to make the trek to Michigan in the summer of 1965, Dewey spent the summer as a park ranger at Whiskytown State Park. The family camped the entire season - spending their days swimming in Whiskytown Lake.

Also in 1965 a new job offer came to Dewey from the school system in Red Bluff, California, just 15 miles south of Cottonwood, so once again the fam-

---

1 *At the time of the move to Northern California, Dewey began using his middle name - Arthur. From then on, he was known in California as Art.*

ily packed up and moved. Within days of moving into their home, Muriel gave birth to their fourth child, Andrew Jon.

Muriel didn't work for almost a year, but when the hospital in Red Bluff needed a '*temporary*' Medical Technologist, she returned to work and continued working there for the next 20 years until her retirement. Even after retirement, she was called back to work at the hospital off and on for several years.

In 1974, Dewey and Muriel moved to a tiny town just east of Red Bluff called Dairyville, where they lived until Dewey's death in 2006. At that point Muriel lived with her daughters until she could no longer walk. She currently resides at a wonderful facility called Red Bluff Health Care.

Muriel and Dewey were married 53 years and have 4 children, 15 grandchildren and 29 great-grandchildren.

"I try to remember always what an old friend of my grandmother's used to say: 'Enjoy every minute you have with those you love, my dear, for no one can take joy that is past away from you. It will be there in your heart to live on when the dark days come.'"

- Eleanor Roosevelt

Additional Resources

Helpful websites:

The Mayo Clinic - *www.mayoclinic.org*
Alzheimer's Association - *www.alz.org*
National Institute on Aging - *www.nia.nih.gov*
A Place For Mom - *www.aplaceformom.com*
AARP -*www.aarp.org/home-family/caregiving*

One particularly helpful and interesting documentary is found on the MUSIC & MEMORY[SM] *site, called "Alive Inside" (http://musicandmemory.org).*
"Film subjects Oliver Sacks and Dan Cohen explain why music acts as a backdoor to memories and shares tips for enjoying music with elders in your life."

Facebook support group:
"www.facebook.com/*Finishing Well for Caregivers*"

Don't be afraid to explore, Google and ask, ask, ask until you get some answers and help.

"It's not where you begin,
it's where you end up."

- Harold Finch, "Person of Interest"
(TV series on CBS)

About The Author

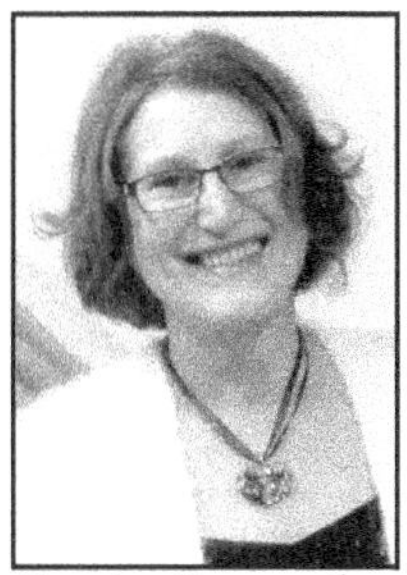

Senia Owensby

Senia Owensby has always loved to write. Her passion for writing has produced a broad variety of literature, including short stories, several children's books, and an assortment of articles for numerous publications.

Her mother's decline into dementia has been a long journey filled with both challenges and joys. She realized that others walking along the same path could benefit from her stories. The purpose of this book was to provide hope for fellow caregivers.

Senia is a Certified Life Coach who lives in a small cottage in Northern California. She's married to the love of her life, and is also a mother and grandmother. When she's not working, she enjoys gardening and writing.

She can be contacted at seniaowensby@gmail.com or through her blog www.finishingwellinlife.com

www.ingramcontent.com/pod-product-compliance
Lightning Source LLC
Chambersburg PA
CBHW021336290326
41933CB00038B/775

* 9 7 8 0 9 9 6 2 9 7 8 0 6 *